MODERN MEDICINE WOMAN: You are the miracle

Published by Gatekeeper Press
2167 Stringtown Rd, Suite 109
Columbus, OH 43123-2989
www.GatekeeperPress.com
Copyright © 2021 by Julyet Berlen

The cover design, interior formatting, typesetting, and editorial work for this book are entirely the product of the author. Gatekeeper Press did not participate in and is not responsible for any aspect of these elements.

ISBN (hardcover): 9781662908408
eISBN: 9781662908415

Front and back cover photography by Elif Koyuturk
Photography by Elif Koyuturk
Food photography by Erkan Yavas
Cover and Book Design by HNBeat Inc.
Edited by Cam "Tink" Daniel

TABLE OF CONTENTS

INTRODUCTION ...6

CHAPTER 1 / Medicine ... 14

Medicine / A Message By Taita Juanito ... 18

"Yage" ...19

Finding The Right Teacher ...20

My Connection With Taita Juanito ...20

The Plant Power / Yage ...29

The Feminine Power ...32

Menstrual Cycle As A Spiritual Path ...32

Cycle Awareness ...33

Dearest Sisters ...33

Moon-Time ...33

How To Use ...34

Yoni Stream ...35

Yoni Egg ...35

Copal ...36

Bitter Bath ...36

Sweet Bath ...36

The Plants ...38

Recipe ...39

How To Prepare For A Plant Ceremony / "Dieta" ...40

Self Respect ...42

Community ...44

Co-Parenting ...44

CHAPTER 2 / The 50/50 ...48

Breathe Into Your Heart ...57

Letting Go ...60

CHAPTER 3 / Creation {rocess ...70

CHAPTER 4 / What is Keto ...78

    What is the Difference Between Keto and Paleo? ...80

    How Did I Start My Keto Journey? ...80

    Let's Talk About Fat ...82

    Staying In Ketosis All The Time Is Not Healthy ...83

    Fitness On Keto ...84

    Sleep ...85

    Here Are Some Tips For Good Sleep ...86

    Meditation ...88

CHAPTER 5 / FASTING ...92

    How Excited Are You To Start? ...94

    Here Is Your New Shopping List: ...99

    Preparation For Fasting ...102

        Journaling ...102

    Why Is Insulin Sensitivity Important? ...105

        What Is Leptin? ...105

        How Does Leptin Work? ...105

        Day 1 ...107

        Day 2-7 ...107

        Day 8-15 ...107

        0-12 Hours ...108

        18th Hours ...108

        24th Hours ...108

        48th Hours ...108

        72nd Hours ...108

    Refeeding After A Prolonged Fast ...109

CHAPTER 6 / Food Is Medicine ...112

    Recipe Index ...115

    Afterword ...146

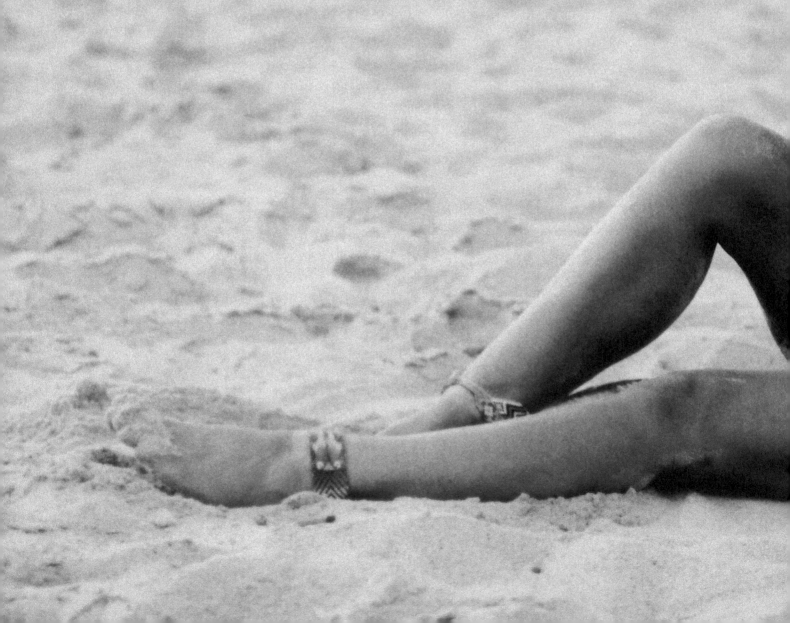

Dedicated to my babies,
Rain and Hunter.

I love you with all my heart.
Mummy.

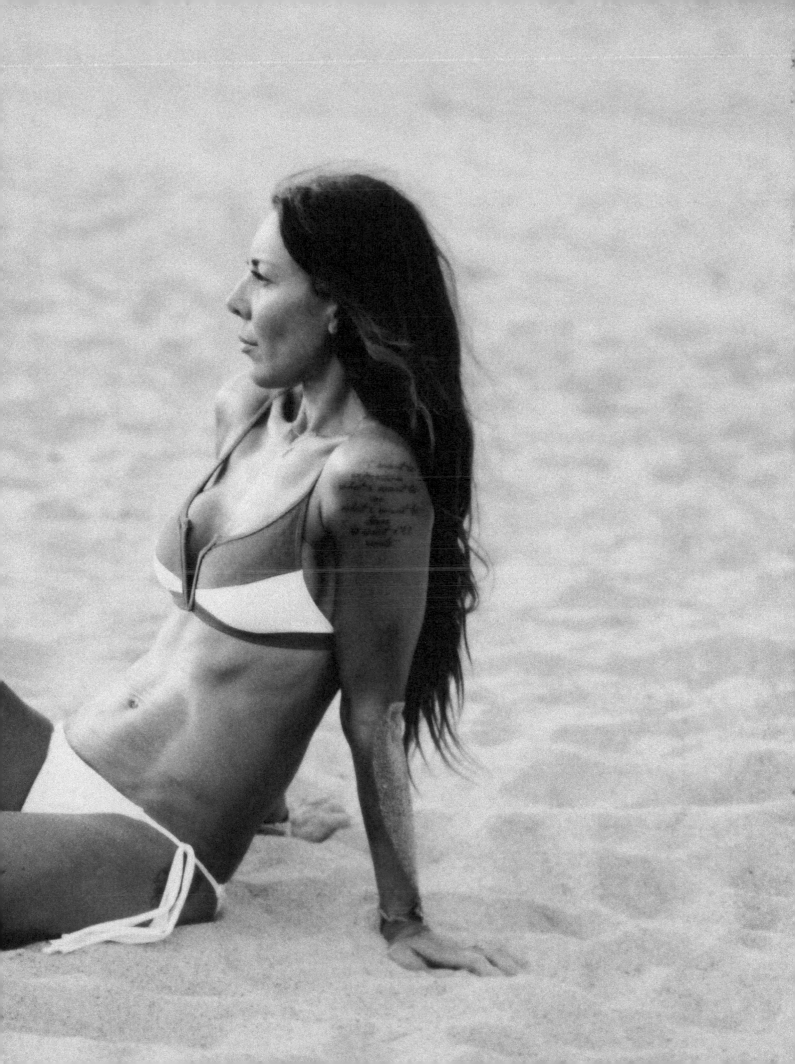

INTRODUCTION

This book you're holding in your hands, as well as all of the information collected and recorded within it, is the story of my personal journey leading up to the life I live now.

I was always the odd kid, black sheep of the family, rebel, definitely not "normal." Nothing ever made sense, up until I found my medicine, YAGE.

YAGE has made an enormous impact in my life, and this whole perspective shift, and feeling the love deeply in every aspect of my life has definitely been the turning point.

I learned the key is LOVE. And I also learned it's hard to LOVE everything and everyone. Before this shift, I didn't love everyone … that's the honest truth. My journey was definitely not easy. Throughout this process I experienced many ups and downs.

Inevitably, I stopped seeking confirmation, validation and approval from outside sources. I learned that the source of everything that is meant to fulfill me is already inside me, and guess what? It's already inside you too. It has been there all along; I just discovered it when I finally learned to look within. I realized the quieter I got, the louder it got, it became more apparent to me everyday.

This is a very personal book, I have seen the real magic in my own life and I have taken great care to detail as much as possible here.

First of all I stopped the blame game. I stopped blaming my parents, blaming the society, blaming how I grew up, blaming the programming, because now I had access to the power within me to change all that. I am the creator of my own reality, and no one is in charge of me but me.

My choices, my decisions, these are what determines my destination. No one else is responsible but me. That was my first lesson to learn. It was also the biggest lesson for me to learn.

Basically, it comes down to owning your own shit. Good and bad. Embrace this moment right here, right now. Feel and feel. What are you really feeling? I know it's hard to get honest with yourself but you can't lie to yourself forever either.

Once you get honest with yourself, you will set yourself free. Wouldn't you love to be free and express yourself exactly as you feel? Of course you would, but first you have to give yourself permission to FEEL.

Feeling is a gift. It is your soul trying to communicate with you. You are not your intellect (mind) you are your heart. Once you tap into your heart things will get hard at first but then you will know you are just flowing and trusting. This is the only way you will be able to liberate yourself from others opinions and words. Nothing will matter enough to change any of what you've become and what you've just discovered within yourself.

"That which you feel yourself to be you are, and you are given that which you are. So assume the feeling that would be yours were you already in possession of your wish and your wish must be realized... so live in the feelings of being the one you want to be and that you shall be."
— Neville Goddard

You are totally in charge, and now you can tap into the abundance, health and wealth that is your birthright.

By connecting to your heart you are remembering who you are, this connection will get stronger; you will go to the origin. What I mean by origin is that, obviously we did not create ourselves, and since we don't really have an explanation for it, a lot of us call this the origin, this energy that runs through our body, "GOD." This energy is in all of us. The source of creation is within us. It is the energy source. The origin that makes our heartbeat and our blood circulate. We have an energy body as well as a physical body. You may also call your energy body your soul, but there is no such thing as only your soul, because you are a soul. You are a soul having a human experience, for a limited time. There is no beginning, no end, we are only passing through this thing we are experiencing called life. Your non-physical body, this energy, this source, is what controls your life, this energy makes us vibrate, it is electricity, that is how we communicate with the universe. And this is all you.

How you feel greatly indicates whether you are in alignment with your source or not. If there is a blockage you will not feel ok, there will be turmoil inside your heart. Your feelings are controlled by your mind. Your thoughts will create how you are feeling and your feelings will create the vibration you are sending out to the

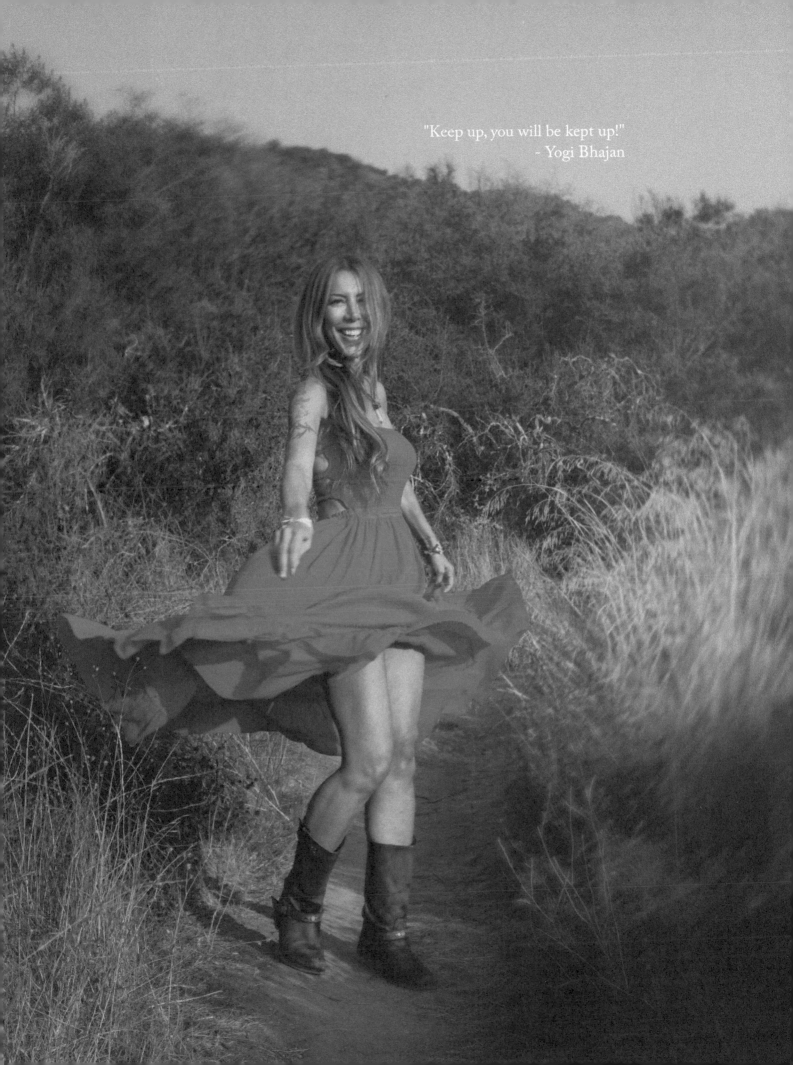

"Keep up, you will be kept up!"
- Yogi Bhajan

universe. Since the universe reflects back what you are putting out there it is most important that you remain aware of your thoughts, of what you're communicating to the universe, GOD the source, whatever the name may be for you, the source within you. Basically the only way you can communicate is by feeling the origin in you, and in order to communicate with the origin, you need to be still and be quiet. This is why meditation is the best tool we have. The entire goal of this human experience is to have joy and to live in unconditional love.

You are not your body; you are not just your five senses. Try closing your eyes and feeling your source. Feel your blood circulating, feel your heart as it beats, feel your skin, and feel your vibration. You are this beautiful being. We are all the same. We are all made by the same source. The same energy. We are alive, that's the miracle and we get to wake up every morning to this amazing human experience, until we don't. Therefore don't let others' opinions take you off your path.

I wrote this book because knowing that we are miracles is not enough. We have to do the work and we have to take care of our physical bodies as well.

Understanding the miracle of yourself and more significantly doing the work to reach your potential with this new knowledge, is what will make you feel better, function better. Personally, I have found that Keto encapsulates all the essentials that allow me to do these things to my highest capacity, because it's all natural, it all already exists in nature and is available to us and consists exclusively of what humans were always intended to survive on. We are not meant to eat food manufactured in factories. We were gifted with all things in nature to let us survive, thrive and heal. I cannot deny the benefits in my own life since discovering keto. I am so passionate about it. I couldn't wait to share it with you. So here we are.

First thing's first, everything starts with self-love and you can't heal the body you hate. Simple as that. Do you love yourself? What will it take for you to take action to better yourself? Do that. Don't wait for others. Don't depend on others, don't be codependent, and most importantly, don't wait to get sick so you can fix it after.

Take care of you while you're still functioning, so your body can keep working for a long time. You don't want to be an old person who is stuck at home or depending on daily medicine intake in order to barely keep surviving. You want to live your best life until your last days. Age truly is just a number. Take care of your heart and your body and they will take care of you. No one will ever love you as much as you love yourself, and no one will ever love you the way that is right for you until you start to do it yourself. It all starts within you.

Believe me, it took me years to learn these lessons. I am sharing them with you in the hopes that it doesn't take you as long as it took me. When the student is ready the teacher appears, they say. I am nowhere near trying to be a teacher but I hope you can see me as a passionate friend who found something that works and I am merely compelled to share it with everyone. It is my purpose, and it is my service to humanity.

If I did it you can do it too. Find what works for you, take what resonates with you from my experiences and implement those things into your life. I broke down everything here for you to understand in a way that will make sense for you as you never know where this journey will take you. Places you never dreamt of arriving.

If you want to see a miraculous transformation inside your physical being, you must shift your focus to super health and super accomplishments. From impossible thinking to thinking anything is possible. You must shift your entire inner world.

You will learn to shift that invisible self called "your mind" from the state of wishing it, to an intention of willingness to pay attention to whatever comes your way. This process will assist you immensely in your journey.

Miracles are an inside job, go there. Create the magic that you seek in your life. That is your only reality.

I love you with all my heart.

Julyet

You were born with potential.

You were born with goodness and trust.

You were born with ideals and dreams.

You were born with greatness.

You were born with wings.

You are not meant for crawling, so don't.

You have wings.

Learn to use them and fly.

— RUMI

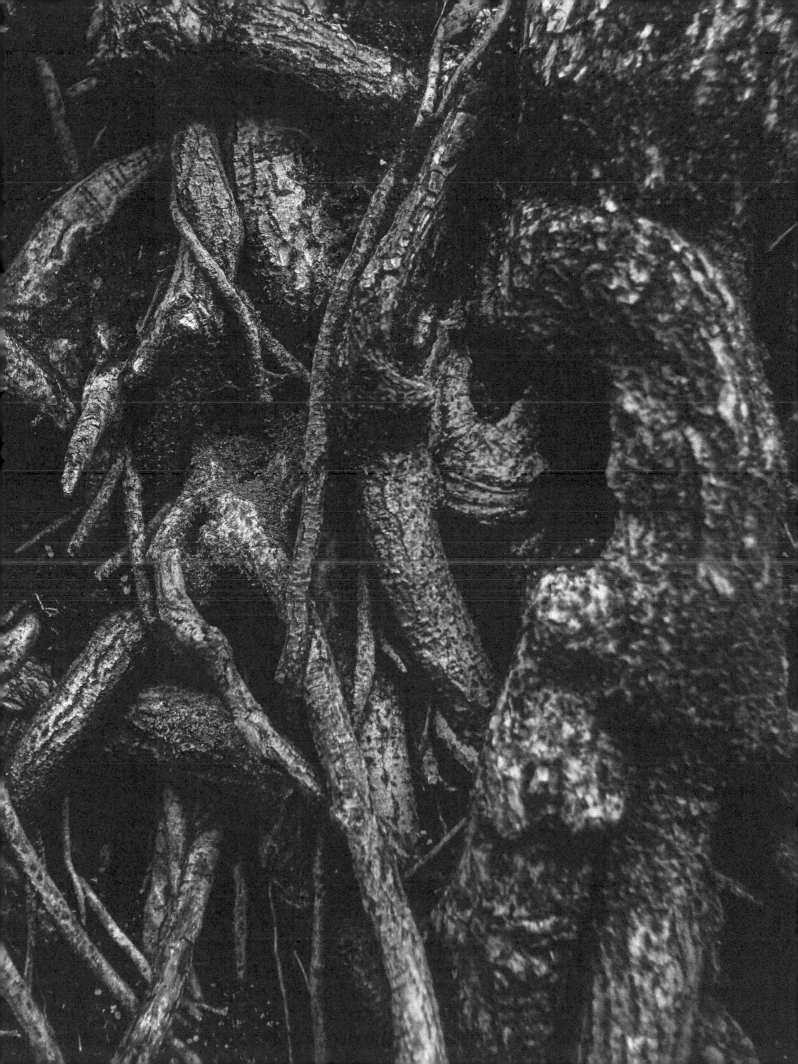

CHAPTER 1

MEDICINE

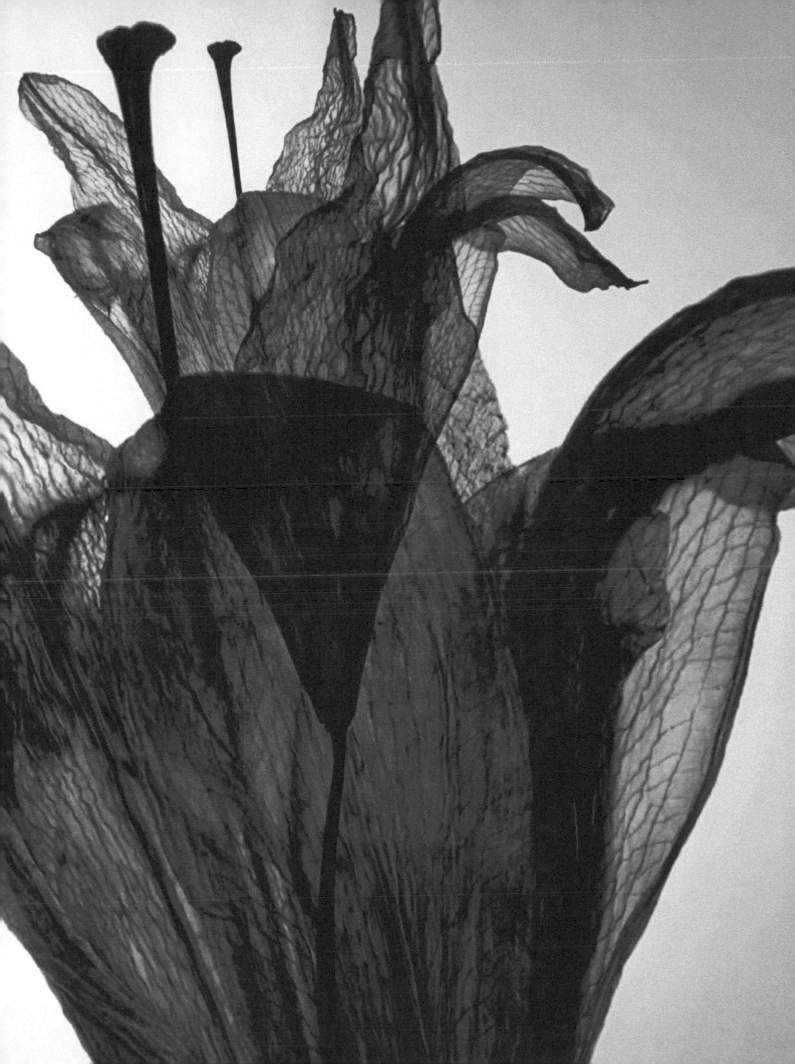

Anything that raises your vibration is a medicine.

Anything that makes you happy is a medicine.

Love is medicine.

Food is medicine.

Music is medicine.

Books are medicine.

Community is medicine.

Nature is medicine.

Animals are medicine.

Plants are medicine.

Friends are medicine.

Children are medicine.

Solitude is medicine.

The Master of all Medicine is the YAGE.

This is my medicine.

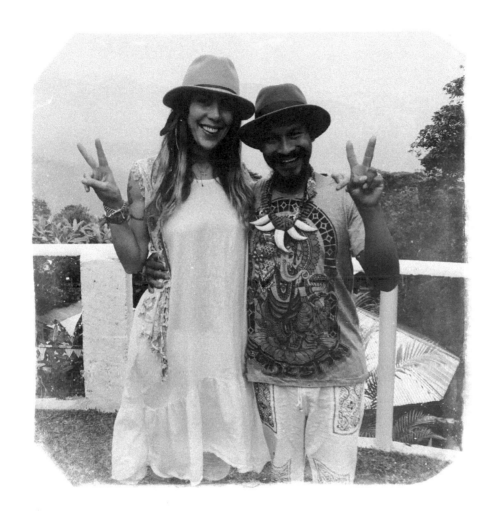

Me & Taita @ Finca

March 22nd - 2018 ♡

MEDICINE
A message by **TAITA JUANITO**

The path towards the awakening of consciousness has carried us to rediscover the ancestral memory through the plants.

The Yagé is a plant of cleaning, of purification, that throughout time has cleansed and offered healing to the human race.

It is a gift from God that has supported us to continue forward on this path towards awakening.

We give thanks to the Great Spirit & to all of nature for guiding us and allowing us to work with these healing plants.

The path of yagé is also about reconnecting with the memory of our ancestors and living in presence.

The path is a long one, and so we must ensure that it is always full of sweetness, compassion, love, & awakening.

TAITA JUANITO

"YAGE"

What is self -care? I love how people think that self-care is only fitness or eating well, or taking hot baths with roses.

I mean those are the side effects of self-care. Yes, I definitely support hot baths with candles and music too. I am all for it.

For me though, self-care starts inside, sitting in quiet and listening to my inner talks first. Being connected to my source, just listening. I actually love sitting in the quiet. I close my eyes and I go. I'm not "meditating" so much as I'm just watching my thoughts. A lot of people may refer to this as meditating but I prefer not to label it. I don't like labels.

Inside of my thoughts, in the quiet I can hear better. It's almost like there is someone else who lives there. That may sound a bit crazy, but if you try it you will see. Your inner voice, it's always talking, sometimes saying things that you would not dare to say out loud.

I started to pay a bit more attention to that voice as I continued this practice. I started making my decisions according to my inner voice. There were a lot of questions I had, and I needed answers. I was stuck, I had no idea what to do, where to go, or with whom to discuss my questions. I only knew that there was something bigger than what I could personally see and hear. I wanted to discover more of this magic. I wanted to connect to that power on a stronger, deeper level. It was like my brain or my heart or both were talking to me. I didn't know which one was which. I didn't know which voice to follow.

I had a lot of beliefs, a lot of rules, OMG the programming I had, and it was not serving me anymore. I was at a point in my life that I was questioning every action I was taking. I was more aware of everything and since I wanted to create my life on my terms and on purpose, I was determined to dive in and go all the way. I was willing to do whatever it took. I was so unhappy, so unsatisfied and nothing made sense anymore. My biggest question was, Why am I here?

This is when I found YAGE, and I found my teacher Taita Juanito. I made a decision and the universe provided. Everything starts with a decision. Everything!

FINDING THE RIGHT TEACHER

For me, No words can describe him, he is poetry in motion!

Taita Juanito is a traditional Inga - Doctor to the indigenous community of the Colombian Amazon, and he walks the path of the Yage (Ayahuasca). His family comes from a long lineage of traditional botanists. Throughout the past 15 years he has been learning and sharing with different communities.

MY CONNECTION WITH TAITA JUANITO

Let me start with when I was first introduced to medicine. I did a lot of in-depth research before I found a safe place to experience the medicine. I wanted to make sure I was not in a jungle somewhere where I didn't feel safe. I am a city girl and not necessarily interested in camping or bugs. I wanted a bit of comfort and luxury. After almost three years of research, I finally came across a place in Costa Rica that had just opened, called Rythmia Life Advancement Center.

This is where my first experience with medicine began. Rythmia was perfect. I recommend this location to anyone who is just starting his or her journey into medicine. As always, of course, consult with your physician before committing to putting anything new into your system. I can only tell you that it was magical for me, I felt pampered, awakened, and I always felt safe.

In my first plant ceremony, I had a vision of this shaman, named Taita Juanito and I was being told: "You need to drink Taita's medicine." I had no idea who he was. I didn't know medicines were prepared differently or that different shamans attributed different energies with different recipes, meaning they added ingredients with certain intentions while preparing the medicine.

As soon as I had the opportunity, I asked Gerry, The founder of Rythmia, "Who is Taita Juanito and what is his medicine? I was told in my journey I need to drink his medicine." Gerry didn't seem to be surprised at all, and replied simply that Taita wasn't there but that I would drink his medicine on Thursday night. "Yage" is what Taita calls his mixture of medicine. He only visits Rythmia four times a year, but his medicine is there all year around. Only served on Thursday nights by the healers who are trained by Taita Juanito himself. Taita Juanito has to give permission in order for someone else to serve his medicine. It is a spiritual contract that he has with the medicine, without his blessing no one can serve his medicine. Medicine belongs to the Mother Earth (Pachamama), and with the utmost respect, the rules need to be followed. You are dealing with the highest energy, with the creative force. Therefore, the healers who are given permission to serve the medicine need to go through a massive training. It takes years and years of study. Learning all this made me feel even safer. I knew I was going to be looked after to the fullest potential.

I still didn't understand all of these concepts back then but I instinctively trusted Gerry and I took his word for it.

Deep down I knew I had to meet this shaman named Taita Juanito, I just felt that he was the teacher for me. I respect people who not just talk but walk the walk.

I had a profound experience at Rythmia, I made amazing friends, I actually cried when the week ended and we said our goodbyes. I didn't want to leave.

I remember it like it was yesterday, as I was waiting for my shuttle to take me to the airport. I went online and found www.fincaambiwasi.com and booked my spot for the next retreat Taita Juanito was holding at his farm in Colombia.

I just experienced something so magical, I knew there was no way I was going to stop, and I needed to go further, to see what else was out there. I knew I had finally found sanity.

After two months of waiting, I was at last flying to Colombia. I remember being so scared at the airport. I didn't speak a word of Spanish back then and I had never been to Colombia. On top of it, I knew no one, I wasn't used to doing things alone, I had been codependent my whole life and at that moment I wasn't sure if they would forget to pick me up. Basically, I was terrified at this point.

But the universe has a way of supporting you when you need it most. Because I made a decision, I was supported by the source, which is how it all works, as long as you trust and surrender, it will never fail you.

On the same flight over I met some other American's (including Joda who still to this day is my best friend). They were flying to Finca Ambiwasi with me and when I found that out, I almost hugged them with joy. I immediately felt safe again, and we connected like we had known each other for years. There was a tangible bond between us. I believe it was Taita Juanito bonding us to each other when we all most needed the support.

After an easy flight we landed. We were picked up and taken to Finca Ambiwasi, which we still call The Farm. It was a two and a half hour drive from the Bogota International Airport. Driving through the city reminded me a little bit of Istanbul, where I was born. Colombia was different than I had created it to be in my head. It was so pleasant, and so raw and so familiar to me. I was home at last.

When we arrived at The Farm I was like a little kid, looking to see this superman, Taita Juanito. Where is he? I wondered. I was so excited to meet him but I could not see him anywhere yet. I was so impatient to meet him and so excited for it. I asked one of my new friends, "Have you seen, Taita yet?"

My friend said, "yes, he just took your suitcase and carried it to your room."

I was like, WHATTTTTTTT? My jaw just dropped and I was thinking, how did I miss that, I was waiting all this time to meet him, and he was just here and I didn't even notice. My jaw was still open and my eyes were popping out, I was still in shock that he took my bags and I treated him like he was one of the helpers at the farm. He looked like a little kid and my friends were laughing at me and of them said, "Close your jaw you will catch a fly."

After the initial shock I calmed down and went to my room. My heart was beating so fast, I have to be honest I was definitely starstruck. Secretly scanning the area to catch him again.

I was blown away, because I had many teachers, gurus, you name it, I worshipped them all thinking they were better than me. Just because I felt I had to be below them so they could teach me. I realized that this belief was implanted in me in the first grade.

I still remember my first grade teacher, she was mean to me, she was very strict with every student but for some reason she was even worse with me. For god sakes, I was only six years old. I got yelled at a lot, I was so scared to go to school because I knew I would be yelled at all day, I was scared to make mistakes on my homework. I didn't want to go to school at all. Finally after I finished third grade my mom changed my school.

In Turkey, from first grade to fifth grade you are with the same teacher. I feel she had a big impact on my insecurity about schooling and teachers, I was like an abused puppy, it took me a good year to get used to my new teacher and to trust her. She loved me but I was not sure if one day she would suddenly become just like my first teacher and thank God She never did.

I only hope my first teacher found happiness somehow, and though there's a good chance that she has passed away by now. I only send her blessings anyway. I forgave her a long time ago. Back then; I felt that I was nobody, just a student, so small and insignificant in this big world, full of bigger people than me.

That was my belief. I had forgotten that these people are also human just like me. I realize now, that due to the trauma of my past, I had been putting all of them on a pedestal, not because they had asked for it, but because I had been making that decision for them. This behavior was coming from feeling inferior to my first grade teacher.

It sounds crazy but I understand now that suffered this kind of trauma during my formative years ended up setting a precedent that would go on for most of my life. Only If I had never gone to the source of the problem and see why I was feeling this way, it took a lot of quiet time to hear the answer.

I made this mistake so many times. I have put Taita Juan on a pedestal before I even met him ... Well, I caught myself this time and I was so proud of myself for it. I wasn't going to repeat my old ways.

When you do that, you are taking the freedom away from someone to be free. You need them to live up to your expectations, and this way, you are just taking their freedom away. Because if they make one mistake, bammmm, they are face down, and you blame them for not living up to the potential that you expect them to live up to.

What a horrible thing to do to someone. But until I experienced this revelation, I didn't know what I was doing. I lost many people in my life like that.

I didn't want to lose Taita, but he showed me, from day one, actually, minute one, he was my equal, he is me, I am him and he is my mirror as I am his, and this goes for everyone around him.

I have never met anyone like him in my life. He says: "Yes, my title is Taita, but I am still a student as well, I am still always learning, we are learning together, we take this journey together."

He never demands respect. He purely gives respect and unconditional love, and that is what he receives in return from all of us. Not with force, but by just being a living example of what it means to live a life of love.

Until I met him, I had never felt heard, loved, or cared for by a stranger. Sometimes we will be a group of sixty-five people, or up to ninety people in the retreats that he holds and we will all get his individual attention. He has the love and the teachings that allow him to do this and it is enough to fill each of us with his undivided attention and acknowledgment despite the number of the crowd.

When I met him for my first one on one consultation, I told him about my experience in the ceremony and what happened, and how I found him, he said, "We don't find the medicine, the medicine finds us when we are ready." He said, "We will drink medicine tonight and see what she shows us and we will organize everything together. He assured me he would be there with me to take care of me when I need him. And he was, he still is, and I know with all of my heart that he will always be and he is. I just close my eyes and connect to my heart and I call him, and there he is. The ultimate WiFi.

When he talks to you and looks into your eyes, you know he is sincere; you have this absolute understanding and certainty. This is a trust I cannot put into words.

I trust him and I no longer put him on a pedestal. No one goes on a pedestal anymore. I see him as someone who dedicated his life to the betterment of humanity, the saving of the Amazon. He lives to serve, to serve this planet, this enormous, worldwide community and despite all that, he is still a father and a husband, a brother and a son. He is part of a family. He is a family man. He is just like you and me. He's just ahead of the game. He is being the light, he is here to guide. He is here to help us remember just who on earth we are.

After knowing all this new information, for as long as I live, I will be in service to mother earth too, and the planet, and I am honored to walk this path with my dear teacher, Taita Juanito. When you find your teacher you will have this feeling in your gut, you will feel exactly how I feel, you won't feel alone anymore.

Keep that person close; keep them in your prayers, in your heart, soul, spirit and staying connected always.

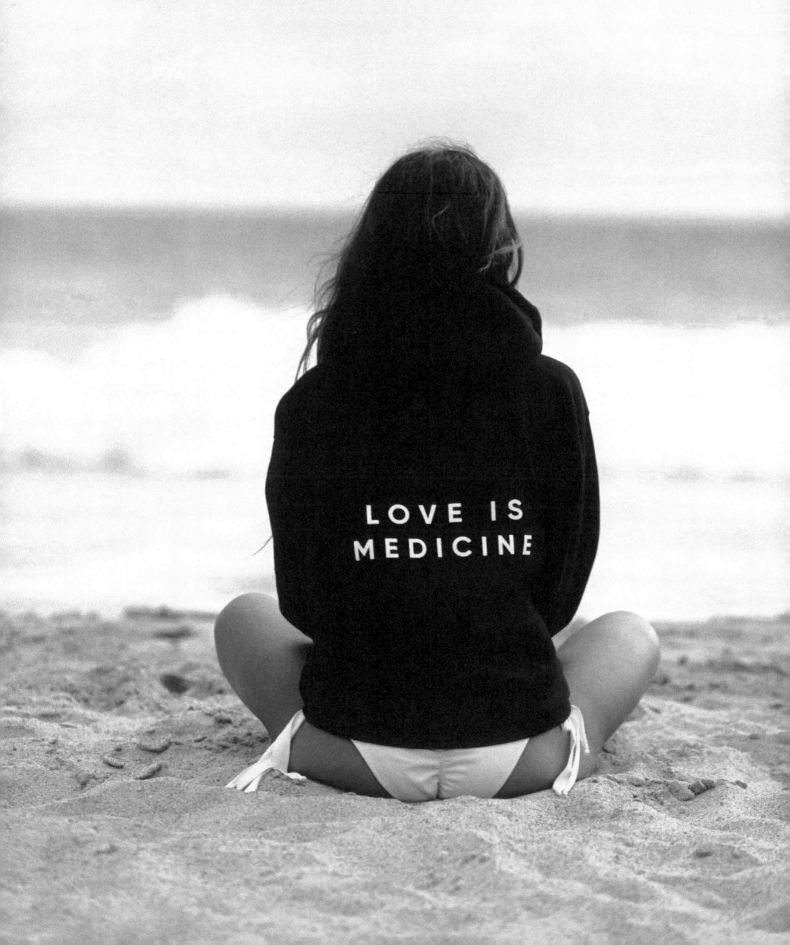

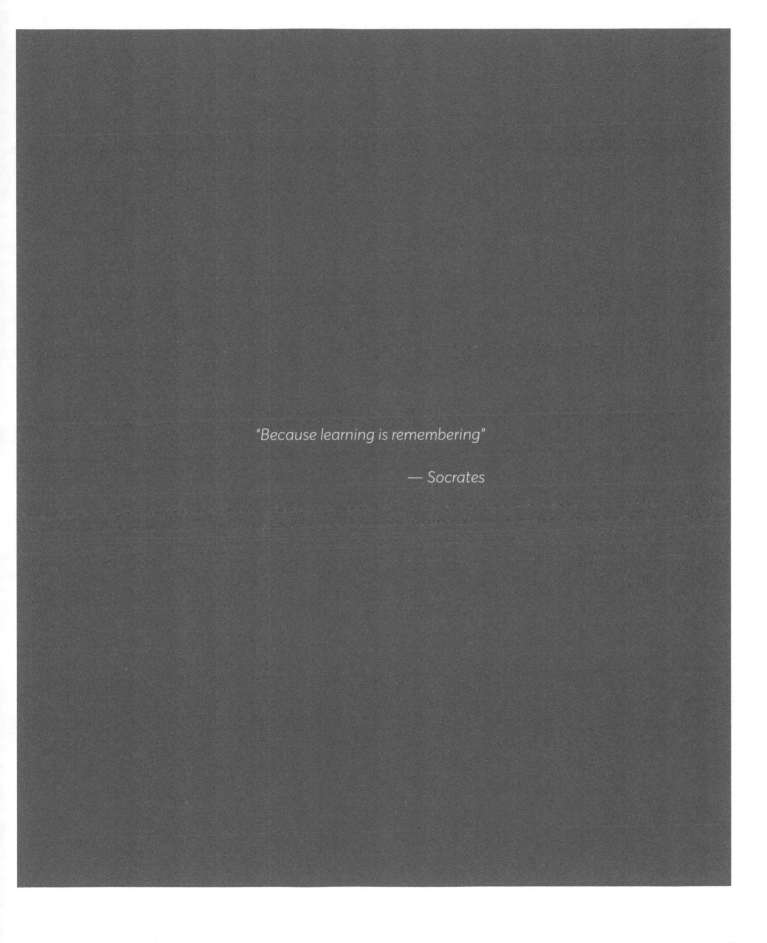

"Because learning is remembering"

— Socrates

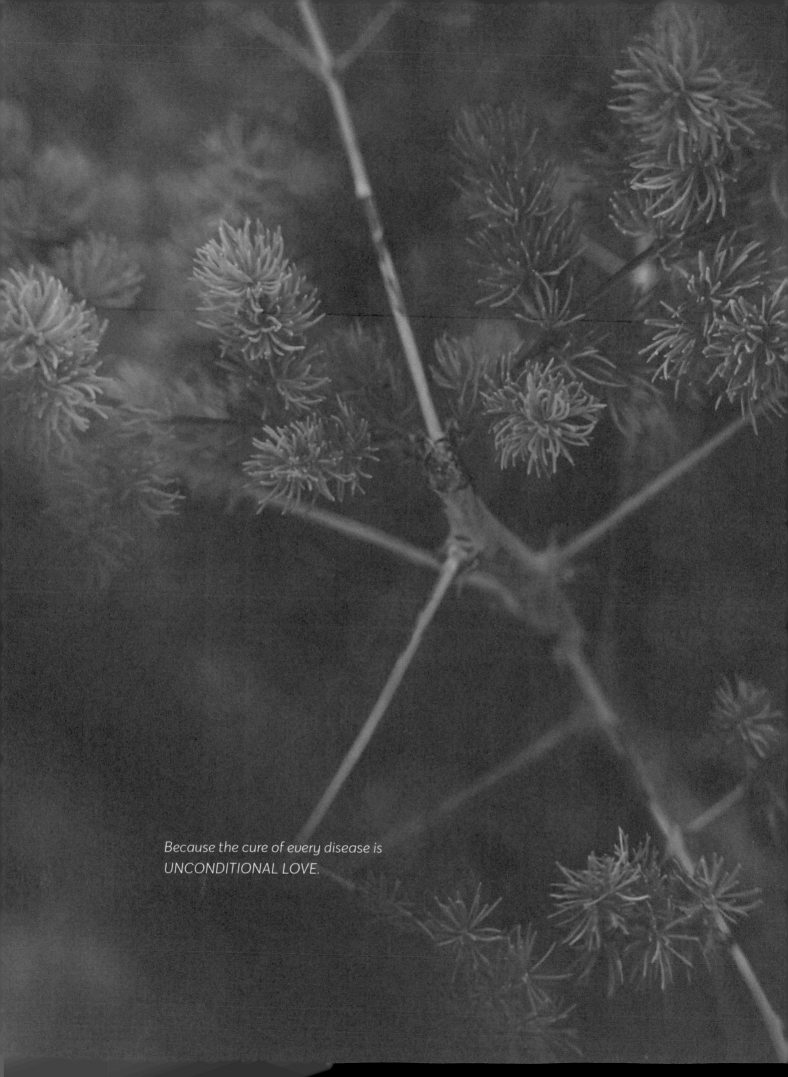

Because the cure of every disease is
UNCONDITIONAL LOVE.

THE PLANT POWER

YAGE

Yage is the medicine that gave me all my answers. It was like opening a can of worms though, not what I was expecting at all. I thought everything I believed was wrong within me and I would be fixed in one ceremony. Tada! Some people do, in fact, experience this. But me, I am a rather complex case, with my luck I probably need 100 more ceremonies. I don't want to say I am a bit thick but I will say that I have a hard time with change. So I push every boundary you can think of.

I found out that we carry in our DNA six generations of karma from our mother and six generations of karma from our father. I was like great. Now what!?! (exclamation-fucking-point!!!)

When you attend a Yage ceremony, you should know, that night may very well be the hardest night of your life, but the sun will always come up in the morning and you'll see it shine as though you've never seen it shine before. You will be made new. Taita says, drinking Yage is like doing 20 years of therapy in one night.

At this point I was like, hmm, maybe I took this self-care business a little too seriously. Can I bail now? But God knew where in Colombia I was. I was in the middle of absolutely nowhere, as far as I could tell. So while I was immensely intimidated by the depths I'd likely be plummeting into, I was more afraid of getting lost in the great wide open of Colombia than doing 20 years worth of therapy in one night...

I thought ok, I came all the way here, left my babies at home with their dads, took time off from work, I went straight up 'off the grid,' like for real, for 10 days. I made a commitment and there is just no bailing missy....

I was ready to clean the pipeline, get a clean slate, live my own life, not my mom's life, not my dad's life I was going to live my life on my terms and I was ready to do whatever it took to get to a point where I would find whatever this new life of mine was going to be.

Since then, I have been a part of over 60 ceremonies, maybe more, I've lost count, and I want to point out that this is not a competition with anyone who has less or more ceremonies under their belt. It's now my lifestyle, it's part of my life, that is the only way for me to stay connected to Pachamama and learn from her but what matters is what happened to me, and inside of me, during the process. We're at a pivotal moment in my story, and you're about to learn what happened to me.

I was able to get rid of so much of the trauma that was in my DNA, I was able to see what I am here to do, I am now only following my heart and trusting my inner voice, it never fails me. Because now I know where the voice is coming from. If it's a feeling from my heart then I am on the right track, but if it's the mind talking then it usually involves some sort of survival component.

When you drink Yage, she will take over, she will go into places that you didn't even know existed. She will scan your body as she travels through it. Our bodies are balls of energy, and energy can get stuck in places that will cause any number of diseases. Yage will unplug all clogged energy, you will feel lighter, you will notice changes in your life. You will start thinking differently and you will start seeing things from a new perspective.

Yage enters your subconscious where there are so many beliefs but your subconscious only delivers the order it gets from your conscious mind, and your conscious mind is clogged by your habits, your programming. The clutter never served you, and somehow, deep in all of us, we already knew this.

Isn't that why you started to look for new ways of changing your life for the better, in the first place? Once you drink Yage, once the veil has been lifted, you will start making new decisions, and you will start sending new orders to your subconscious, and your subconscious mind has no judgment but to deliver what you believe, because you tend have feelings attached to what it is that you believe to be true for you. Once you get the hang of that, you will be in charge of your life. That is what Yage gives you. This is the formula to creating your own life the way you want to design it. You are the creator. So how aware are you of your thoughts, beliefs, and feelings?

If you believe it, and feel it, you will see it. Period!

So I believe "self-care" is taking care of your inner self first. Once you do that, then the meditation, yoga, hot baths, long walks, mani-pedi's follow! I love doing all of that, by the way. I actually look forward to time alone, to simply take it all in.

Life is so beautiful, I feel so blessed that I get to wake up every morning, and when I realize that I'm up, I am filled with joy, I am very happy that I'm awake, awake to live and play another day. I think of how many people didn't get to wake up in the morning, I look at my kids, and see that they woke up too, bam, another win, my kids are up. It's that simple for me, that's self-care for me, I am so grateful for the things I have in my life, most of all to have my health.

I am not telling you to book a trip to Colombia right this moment to experience the ceremonies and drink Yage. Though, if that's what you're doing, wow, you don't waste time, and good for you! In all seriousness, though, Yage is just a tool, a productive and powerful one, yes, but it is just one way to reach the deepest parts of your heart. I am sharing my experience with you so you can make your own decision and see what path you want to take. You will find what works for you. You have already come so far.

When you are ready you will know, you will be wondering, you will be googling things, you will start questioning. I mean you bought this book didn't you? If you were looking for a sign, you are holding the sign in your hands. That's how medicine found me and maybe medicine will find you, when you are ready and it's your journey, she will find you, too.

If you do feel the call to go in the direction with Yage, you can always do your own research and ask Doctor Google.

You can also go www.fincaambiwasi.com to see if that's something you are ready to do. Dive in, and embrace the knowledge that once you go that way there is no going back and there will be no desire to either.

Are you ready to take the RED PILL?

Now let's talk about other ways of self-care. Sleep, meditation, long hot baths, nature walks, time with community, time with your children the list goes on and on.

THE FEMININE POWER

In my spiritual journey I have met many amazing souls. They started the journey way before me and now their mission in life is to share what they have learned from elders, from our teachers.

I keep my sisters and brothers close to me, I communicate, I ask for advice, and it has been most helpful. When you know you need help and that it's ok to ask for it, and know that it's always available for you, that is a game changer. I know it was for me.

As I was starting out, I had many questions and I wanted to do everything right, so I asked and in return I got a lot of support. I was given what I needed to grow into and embrace what has given birth to a second nature within me, and now it just flows, it's just a part of me.

My dear sister Yara explains how the moon time is so important in connecting to the divine power of creation. I learned most of this valuable information from her, so I asked her if it's ok for me to share her knowledge and of course the answer was yes.

I am so honored to share this with you and hope you find something that resonates within the connection to the magical creative power within you, as this is available to all women.

This is taken from www.sumakallay.com with the permission of Yara and Michael.

MENSTRUAL CYCLE AS A SPIRITUAL PATH

Embracing myself as a woman has brought the greatest change in my path of healing. This loving acceptance of myself has blossomed from being reminded of long forgotten feminine teachings. When I first heard this wisdom I knew in every cell of my being for it to be true. It instantaneously changed how I saw myself in this world. Because of this, it brings me so much joy to share this forgotten information with my sisters. I truly believe as we embrace all that it means to be a womban we step deeper into our power and bring great healing to ourselves, our loved ones and the world. We do this work in deep reverence for our mothers, grandmothers and all those women that walked before us. We do this work for the generations of women that will follow.

As a woman we each have structured within us a guide to our own healing: the textbook to our spiritual path. We need only connect to ourselves to discover all of creation. Nature has blessed us with the extraordinary ability to bring life from spirit into this earthly world, housing and growing within our womb the miracle of new life. Nothing is more powerful or spiritual than that.

Walking a spiritual path is a study of life, ignited by a curiosity of purpose and desire to live in the most beautiful of ways. As a woman we have an opportunity to experience this study of creation through our menstrual cycle. Once we begin to understand, respect, appreciate and see the magic in our own natural rhythms, we sink deeply into ourselves, our intuition, our creativity, and elements of nature and to each other. We re-learn how to love and accept our sisters, mothers, our grandmothers and ourselves.

We step deeper into our power as a woman, and unveil our unique talents and passions. We restore our connection to the great cosmic uterus, divine mother, divine father and all of creation.

Cycle Awareness

Start by bringing awareness to the ebbs and flows of your monthly cycle. Discover the different phases of energy and emotions you pass through on a monthly basis. In her book "Wild Power," Alexandra Pope describes these phases as the four seasons of the year. Winter being our time of hibernation and bleeding, followed by Spring, emerging slowly from the temple of moon time, into Summer, a time of increased excitement and energy of ovulation, followed by Fall, the preparation for winter, our time of bleeding. Each season comes with its unique energies and is experienced uniquely by each woman. Understanding ourselves in this way brings patience, acceptance and love for ourselves.

Dearest Sisters

Be still, be silent and hear the ancient whispers, calling us to remember our relationship with our menstrual cycle, our moon-time and our sacred blood.

Moon-Time

The essence of the moon time ceremony is experiencing ourselves as divine beings of nature. To feel deeply in our being the power and privilege it is to be a womban in this life. It is a time to explore ourselves as creative beings, to listen to ourselves, our intuition and what we truly need to care for ourselves and be well. It is a time to cleanse, purify, heal and let go of anything no longer serving. It is a time of clear connection with the divine mother, the great uterus and divine father. It is a time to connect deeply with our earth mother, communing with her, learning with her. It is a time to honor ourselves as the powerful women we are, in our own unique way. This ceremony is your own, unique as you. Listen to yourself, trust yourself and enjoy the self-love-affair.

Once a woman starts bleeding the portal to the celestial skies is open and her moon time ceremony commences. Alternatively for women who do not bleed, the full moon represents their time of deep connection and power. Just as the moon is complete and full so are their cycles of bleeding in this life. The more time and space you can create for yourself during this time, the better. Time to be in meditation, prayer, self-reflection, self-care and creativity.

If possible, let go of some of your usual responsibilities, honor this time and your healing process. It is a time of great power, creativity, cleansing, purification and prayer. If your life circumstances don't allow you to take this space, it is ok, this is your life, your prayer and your ceremony, revise it to flow harmoniously with your life. A good practice to start is by giving yourself some time in the morning as well as in the evening for reflection, prayer and self care.

How To Use

The blood we shed has the ability to nourish new life. As our cycle progresses through the month a nutrient dense home is built lining our uterus. If an egg is fertilized it implants itself in this uterine lining and nourishes life into being. If a fertilized egg does not implant itself this lining is released in the form of our monthly blood. This blood is filled with enough vitamins and minerals to nourish life. It is also imprinted with a month's worth of experiences, energies and emotions. Bleeding is a process of cleansing and cleaning all the happenings of our personal lives, the lives of our brothers and sisters and the life of the planet. This monthly cleansing allows us to truly learn how to heal ourselves. This healing happens through our reconnection with nature and mother earth by giving her our blood. Giving this vital information back is a calling home to our earth mother to let her know how we are doing, this way she knows what we need and can help us heal and grow. Our earth mother happily takes all that needs to be released.

When we connect with our earth mother, listen to her subtle ancient wisdom, we step deeper into our harmonious, divine & natural essence.

Yoni Steam

A Yoni Steam, also known as a vaginal steam, or bajos, is the ancient practice of sitting or squatting over a steaming pot of water infused with herbs. It's a powerful ally for female vitality in nourishing the womb, pelvic floor, hormone rebalancing, and cleansing the womb of toxins/trauma/female reproductive illnesses. It is supportive to overall reproductive health and fertility and works as a nourishing ritual for reconnecting a woman with her body and feminine center.

Important: It is not recommended to steam if you have an IUD or during menstruation. DO NOT STEAM IF YOU ARE PREGNANT OR THINK YOU MAY BE PREGNANT.

› www.fourvisionsmarket.com

Yoni Egg

For over two thousand years, wise women across cultures and traditions have used the ancient powers of crystal eggs to bring forth wellness and vitality of the Goddess. Nourishing and strengthening the sexual powers enhance and strengthen the spiritual energy in the body. These crystal eggs are designed to help you to tap into your sensuality and become more deeply empowered in your sexuality. This set includes 3 pieces of different sizes for you to have everything you need to get started. It is suggested to start with the largest stone and as you strengthen your pelvic muscles work towards the smaller one which is the most advanced practice.

Cultivate the sacred energy of love and recharge your heart chakra with the Rose Quartz yoni egg. Reawaken trust through the soothing vibrations to calm and cleanse your auric field to open yourself up to a deeper love connection. The vibration of love that flows from this stone penetrates deeply into the cellular level where it brings harmony and unity to your heart.

This Rose Quartz vaginal stone can transform both intimacy and orgasmic pleasure as it fosters a strong connection between your heart center and your inner sex goddess by releasing wounds, building trust, and activating your spirituality. This soft pink stone infuses a deep healing and rejuvenating energy that inspires you to always act from a space of love, compassion and sensuality.

› www.fourvisionsmarket.com

Copal

This is one of my favorite tools. I use it daily, it is definitely energetically stronger than sage, although I use sage as well, copal is like vacuuming the house with Dyson.

Copal is an ancient resin used throughout the Americas in sacred practice and ceremony. This white copal comes from the Amazon jungle of Colombia. It is hand harvested in prayer and reverence by local tribes. Use it in good consciousness to:

- Bless yourself, your living space, your workspace and your clients
- Ward off negative energy and call in the protection of Light beings
- Energetically protect and purify people, places and spaces
- Draw in the frequencies of tranquility and balance
- Sacred ritual and ceremony to deepen spiritual connection
- Consecrate and anoint artifacts and places
- Awaken and rejuvenate ancestral communications and connections

Application: Can be used directly on the skin for direct protection and blessing or add a few drops in a spray bottle with water to energetically protect your home, workspace, car, sacred items or jewelry. Can also be burnt over charcoal.
› www.fourvisionsmarket.com

Bitter Bath

After a sweet bath, I would also do bitter baths to balance the energy. Usually three days straight sweet bath, a day off, followed by three days bitter bath.
Use this Indigenous plant technology to extract bitterness from your life and offer protection. All you need to do is boil a big pot of water and pour in the bitter herbs, letting it simmer for about an hour. Take off the pot and let cool, and then strain the tea. To apply, use one cup of bitter bath every time you shower. Towel dry and then pour the bitter bath over your body and let it air dry, allowing the plants to seep into your pores. Do this with prayer & intention, calling forth the power of the bitter plants to heal & help you to release pain, trauma, and bitterness.
› www.fourvisionsmarket.com

Sweet Bath

There are times when the energy of life is so dense and heavy for us and things can become too difficult to deal with as they arise. In some Amazonian cultures, they would call this bitterness. Bitterness can increase in your energy from various things like dealing with difficult situations, making hard decisions, having sickness in the body, or participating in any ceremonial activities that may induce the purging, or removing, of old energies.

This bitterness is normal and is a part of a natural cycle of life going constantly from sweet to bitter to sweet and back to bitter again; an eternal balancing act. In order to remove this heaviness, this bitterness, from us, we have to provide something to replace it: sweetness!

Enter plant technology. Land plants have been around for a long time, about 500 million years, and they have been evolving ever since. There is so much we can learn from plants. At some point, some of these plants generated something entirely new to the Earth: sweetness. It began as a way to lure certain insects to come close and take the plants pollen with it when it leaves, a way to reproduce for the plant. After all, the plant cannot move enough to pollinate its neighbors. It needs the help of another part of nature so it can continue to evolve and thrive.

When we speak of incorporating sweetness into our life and our body through sweet bath, the goal is to tap into this energy. We are using the plants to help us the same way the plant used the bees to help them. We offer our intention to the plant and the Earth, that we may draw upon this sweetness to aid us in our continued evolution.

The Plants

When using plants for a sweet bath, the best ones to use are fresh and organic. You could use dry plant materials, but fresh is much better. In the drying process some of the sweetness is lost, so do yourself a favor and find fresh plant matter.

The core plant in any sweet bath will be basil. The intense sweet smell you find in a fresh bundle of basil is haunting, which is what we are looking for. With only basil you can make an incredible sweet bath, however, with some other sweet plants to accompany the basil we can make a bath that is absolutely bursting

Use this recipe as a guideline when making your own sweet bath. The proportions of plants and water and time can all be changed a little and will still create a great sweet bath. This is simply how we do it and we have found it works great.

Needed:

Large stockpot
Strainer
1 bundle Basil
1 bundle Spearmint
1/2 bundle Rosemary

1. Fill the stockpot with 4 quarts of water, all the plant matter, and place on the stove over high heat.
2. When water begins to boil, add the lid and reduce heat to simmer and set the timer for 20 minutes.
3. After 20 minutes, remove from heat and let it cool for 1 hour.
4. After it has cooled to room temperature, strain the plant matter from the liquid.
5. Pour sweet bath into jars or bottles and store in the fridge.
6. Enjoy!

Notes

The sweet bath will stay good in the fridge for about a week. To prolong the life of the sweet bath you could add some alcohol such as vodka at a rate of 1 cup per 4 quarts of sweet bath. This will allow the bath to stay fresh outside the fridge for up to a week, or inside the fridge for several weeks.

Boiling the plant matter for too long will cause some of the sweetness and some of the volatile phytochemicals to be lost. Boiling for 20 minutes and allowing to cool for an hour will ensure a good extraction and that nothing is lost unnecessarily. If the plant material is dissolving and falling apart when you strain, you have boiled too long.

If you are adding other plants that require cooking longer, such as vines and barks, begin with those plants first and add the basil, rosemary and spearmint at the end, 20 minutes before you are done.

How to Use

To use the sweet bath, begin by taking a shower as you normally would. When you are finished showering, dry off normally. You can then apply the sweet bath all over your body. Make sure to apply it everywhere, while also remembering why you are doing it and placing your intention there. The plants work on their own, but your intention activates them to work more precisely and thoroughly.

Allow the sweet bath to air dry on your skin. It is important to allow at least a few minutes for the bath to air dry and absorb into the skin before you dry yourself.

HOW TO PREPARE FOR A PLANT CEREMONY "DIETA"

Here we go. This is one of the most important parts of your healing journey. How we prepare for a plant ceremony literally alters the amount of benefits you will receive during and after the ceremony. The more prepared you are, the greater the results will be, I cannot emphasize this enough.

What you are about to encounter is a very serious business, and not to take it lightly, you are going to be entering new dimensions. How you prepare for a ceremony will help your experience to be the ultimate level. You want to get the best out of this experience and not sabotage it. Here I share my personal preparations. I hope this finds you the best way.

I start my preparations about ten days before.. First of all it starts with my diet. What we are putting in our bodies has a massive effect on the results.

I will cut red meat all together, because the animals before slaughtered feel fear. They release toxins and these toxins stay in their system. This is why it is so important to pick humanely treated animals regardless. I don't want this energy to come out while I'm in a ceremony, because it belongs to the animal.

MODERN MEDICINE WOMAN | MEDICINE

I will usually stick with fish at this time, but three days prior to ceremony I will cut out all animal products. At this time, I usually will be fasting. I will have one meal a day, which will be super light. And the day before the ceremony I will fast all day, no food at all. The day of the ceremony I will have a very light breakfast. One kind of fruit would do. I prefer melons, or pineapples. I will just drink water all day (unless you want to see the food you had at lunch, then you can eat). This is usually my food intake prior to ceremony time. Most people also will cut coffee intake. I have my morning coffee always, because my body is used to it, this doesn't affect me in a bad way.

It is so important to also cut any kind of hot spice and salt intake, this is important, because hot spices and salt will not allow you to have visions (pinta).

Three days prior to ceremony, you can implement sweet baths to clear the energy, and this will bring sweetness into your life. Absolutely NO alcohol, NO sex for at least three days before and after. Sexual energy is a creative energy and it needs to be contained within the body because you will need this energy during the ceremony to heal.

If you are on any kind of medications, you need to check in with your doctor before attending a plant ceremony. Unfortunately you won't be allowed into a ceremony unless you have a clearance from your doctor. Most mind altering drugs will interfere with the plants. You will need to be off of them at least 28 days or more. This also goes for smoking marijuana or taking mushrooms.

You are about to be working with the master plant YAGE therefore you don't want to interfere with it. Your body and mind needs to be a clean vessel for the healing to take place.

YAGE won't be able to enter if you are putting roadblocks on its way. The cleaner and the lighter you are, the easier and most effective the ceremony.

And for the ladies, if you are on your moon you won't be able to attend a YAGE ceremony. The reason is that when we are on our moon we are energetically very powerful and our portal is open to receive, we can take over the room, meaning, since our portal is open, it is never a good idea to do the energy work, we will be receiving all the negative and positive energy all together, this is the reason TAITA won't allow women to attend a ceremony is to protect us. At this time it's a good idea to stay in silence and meditate, reflect, not to do many physical activities. Stay with it and honor this time. And for some reason if you receive your moon during a ceremony, the healers will take you out of the main Maloka (where the ceremony takes place) and place you in the Moon Maloka (it's reserved for the women only for this reason) so you can continue your journey there, there are assigned women healers who will help you during this time. You will never be left alone. This actually happened to me once but now I always make sure I don't plan on attending ceremonies around my moon time.

This is pretty much it, if you prepare whole-heartedly, your experience will be amazing. Life changing. Literally.

SELF RESPECT

These are some nurturing practices I learned from Wayne Dyer.

- Look into a mirror, make an eye connection with yourself and say " I LOVE ME" as many times as possible during your day. I love me, these three magic words will help you maintain your self respect, saying these words may be difficult at first because of the conditions you have been exposed to all your life, but still say it without embarrassment, say it proudly. I LOVE ME.
- Write the following affirmation and repeat it over and over to yourself. I AM WHOLE AND PERFECT AS I AM. By basically carrying these words with you and feeling them, their energy will flow directly to you.
- Remind yourself that you are never alone.
- Respect your body
- Meditate and stay in conscious contact with your source (heart).
- Be in the state of gratitude.

Self-Love

When you are focused on bettering yourself, you learn to hold space for others, because you understand the journey. Everyone's path is different. We are all trying to reach our full potential. Have compassion for others and the energy of love. When we do that, we become more available to serve others. When you take care of your body, you have strength and energy to move through, push

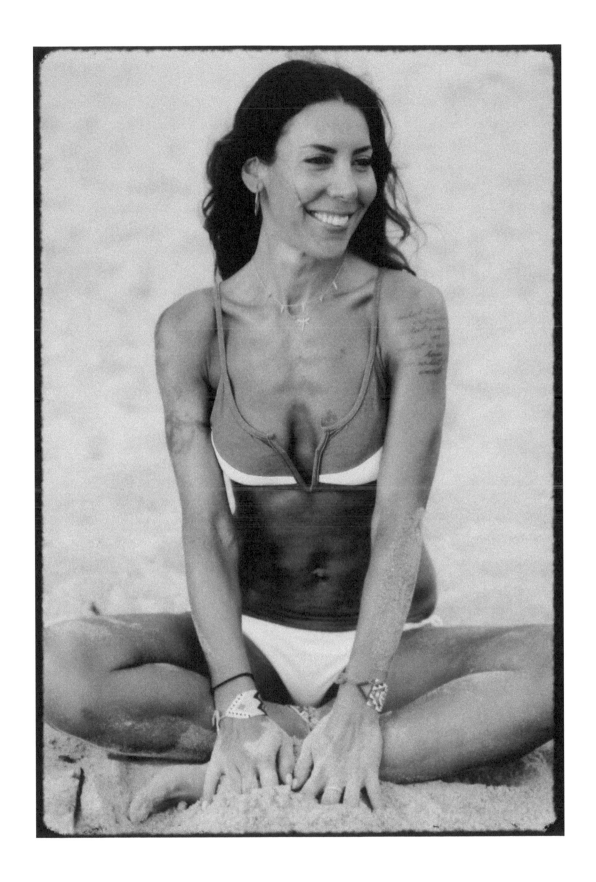

forward. Your body is your vehicle. When you take care of it life gets exciting and more enjoyable.

Self-love and acceptance are everything. It is a hard concept to get used to and you may feel selfish but once you realize you are happier and healthier and that you are serving the ones who are around you with your well being, it changes everything for the better.

> *"You must learn to look beyond the mirror. You are the spirit. You are the self. You are the honor.*
>
> *You are the source of all sources, you are the redeemer of all redeemers.*
>
> *From this creation is born."*
>
> *- Yogi Bhajan*

Community

Like-minded friends are everything, once I found my tribe, they became more like family, maybe even closer than family. It is so good for your soul to have friends who accept you the way you are, nothing more, nothing less. Real friends are treasures to me. They are a big, HUGE part of my happiness.

I say, the life worth living is the one where you can be you.

Co-Parenting

I am a single parent by choice and I used to have a really bad out look before sharing my babies with my ex's.

After YAGE, even that changed for me. I lost my possessive ways with my kids. I started seeing more of what they needed. I was able to go beyond my ego and my own needs.

I started putting their needs and wants first. I asked myself, if I were a kid what would I want? I would want my parents to be involved equally. I would want to be loved and cared for by both parents, not because my parents were fighting over me and I had to choose which one to love more, or where I would spend more time

All this competition between parents, it puts a lot of pressure on children. They feel quilt and they feel they are always doing something wrong. That is not how I want to program my kids. They are free.

So I dropped the nonsense as a parent and started sharing my kids with their dads more. I let them have a relationship, and with that came the opportunity to make memories. I came to realize and accept that, just because I gave birth to them, it didn't mean I OWN them more than their dads do.

Again, I'm doing me, I am not telling anyone what to do, not by any means. These are just my tools to stay stress free. It is self-care.

The best thing to give,
Your enemy is forgiveness,
To an opponent is tolerance,
To a friend, your heart,
To your child, a good example,
To your father, deference,
To your mother, conduct that will make her proud of you,
To yourself, respect,
To all men, charity.

– Wayne Dyer

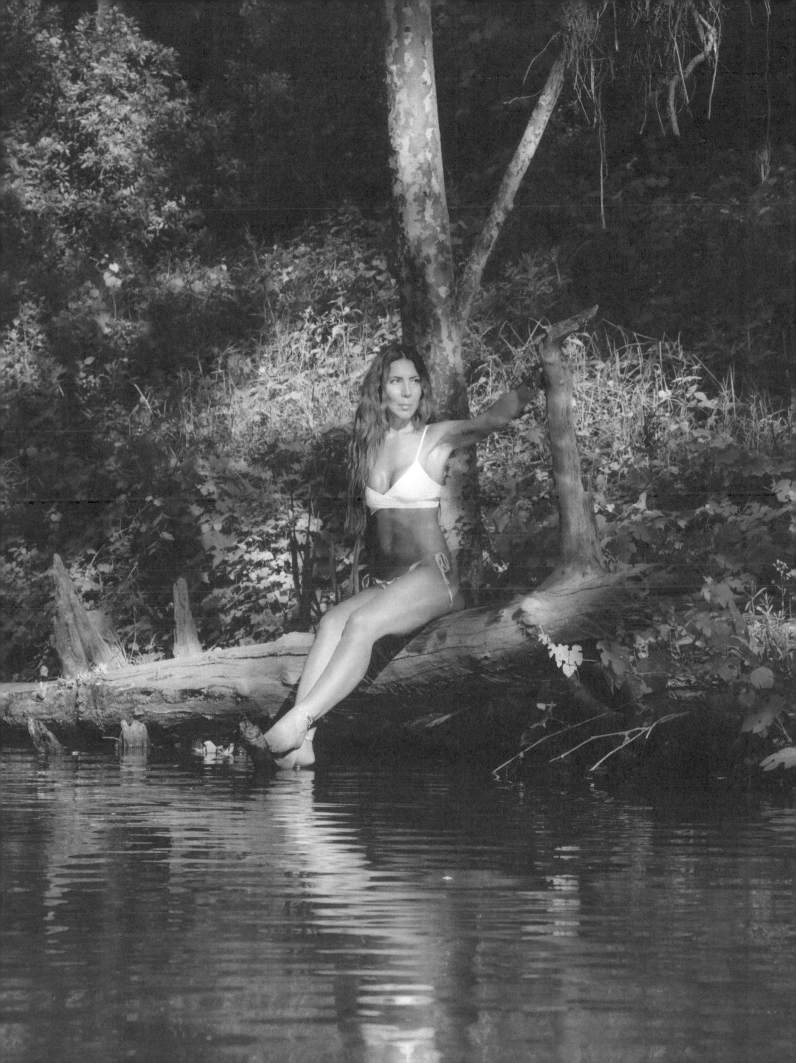

CHAPTER 2

THE 50/50

THE 50/50

My teacher Taita Juanito always talks about the 50/50. He says, "the medicine will do the 50% but the other 50% is up to you."

What he means is this. When you drink medicine, medicine will do the cleaning, lifting of the veil, healing of the body, healing of emotions, and it will give you a clean slate to start over.

Then the integration process starts. There will be a lot of reflecting, reflecting on how you were before and how you are after. Now with your new perspective, nothing will be the same, the things you were ok with before won't make sense, you will look back at certain things and say, "Wow, I can't believe I said yes to that," or "I can't believe I said no to that." Your standards just become higher. You wake up. Welcome to life ☺.

In this process of change, you will have the urge to take care of your body and mind more diligently. You will begin a journey of enlightenment and begin to understand that ultimately, it's your well-being that is most important. You being well is where being well being starts. Once you learn and accept this information as your ultimate truth, no obstacle will land in your path that you won't willfully and peacefully be able to overcome.

You will eat better, you will move more, you will meditate, and you will make more time for yourself.

You will start saying no easily to things you were not able to turn down before, or yes to things that now resonate within you without hesitation. You will start making decisions with your heart more. Attempting to please others won't even cross your mind the way they once did. Let's be honest, I am sure you said yes to many things, just to avoid conflict. I know I did.

I was always making sure people around me came first. I wanted to make sure everyone liked me, I never wanted to rock the boat, ever, and I lived my life trying to avoid all conflict. The cost was not being true to myself. That was so not healthy, it literally ate my soul up slowly and the damage was so obvious when I finally had my eyes opened. I believe that is why I hit rock bottom. I stayed in wrong relationships, made way too many mistakes. But those are mistakes that today I'm grateful for, because of the depth of how much I learned.

I can tell you now, never again. My first time after I started doing medicine, I was sitting in awe, watching what was unfolding, it was so new to me, I was a bit lost, like learning to walk again, so many habits I had to break, rewire myself again. I learned to ask for help from those who have walked this path before me. Once you get involved with a community of like-minded people you will never feel alone again.

You meet so many amazing souls who are more than willing to hold your hand, teach you how to walk again. I was and still am so blessed to have my Finca Ambiwasi family, my new family; we were and still are, all in this journey to remember together.

I moved to the USA at age 24, I have been alone ever since, I have no family members here, just me, the black sheep. It was my choice, so I never hold them responsible for my loneliness here, or lack of family support. I had a big mission ahead, and deep down I knew I was going to do it, with them or without them. I remember the day I became a citizen, I remember crying so much with so much pride (if you are an immigrant reading this, you know what I am talking about).

After a long time always working and trying to make it in America, I forgot to take care of the most important part, my heart. I was in my head all the time, always in survival mode. Massive, masculine-energy driven Julyet. I became a go-getter, get it done, just do it. If you don't do it no one will do it for you. This is what I was taught along the way.

Now when I look back, I am so grateful for every burden, every challenge, and every win. I appreciate everything, because of all that I went through, I am here today. I did it alone, and I am proud of it.

I love my life now, I love that I have two amazing babies, I love that I am able to write this book, I love that I get to live in an amazing place. I am free to do anything I want, no limits to my imagination.

Finding plants was my miracle. I deserved it. I got it, thank you, universe ☺.

After you find yourself, you really want to live fully, life truly is so short, and I want to make the best of it by being super healthy, fit, gorgeous and happy.

Yes you can be all. Why would you limit yourself?

Live in your full potential, life is short. One day I was listening to Tony Robbins, whom I study religiously explained it perfectly; I will share it with you here:

Someone asked him, how do you balance your life?

He said, "I don't. I don't believe in it." When I heard that I was like, OMG I thought I was weird, because that's exactly how I think as well.

Then he explained, "think of a seesaw, and you balance it, now your work life and personal life is even, balanced. You are hanging in the air, perfectly balanced. How long can you stay like that? You will be bored out of your mind. It's not fun, you will have an urge to go up and down, and up and down. Isn't that the whole point of a seesaw, that's where the fun is."

He explained further with these words, "I really think balance is more about integration, how do I make sure the areas in my life, like my wife, my kids, my companies, my health, how do I balance that? I do streaks, I do intense work, then take intense total time off, spend time with my family. Work intense, play intense. Take total time off. So when I do each task in front of me I am totally in the present moment and I enjoy it."

Ahhhhh, such a breath of fresh air! This is exactly what I have been doing for years, minus the taking time off for vacations. I work and I spend time with my kids, but taking total time off is on my bucket list, when I am like Tony Robbins, I promise I will do that too ☺.

I am a passionate person, I do everything with a lot of intensity, I play many roles. I am a mother, I am a medicine woman, I am a hairdresser, I am a holistic health coach, I am a fitness instructor. I have many hats, and I love them all. Now, I am an author as well. This passion for writing I've had all my life, this is my dream true. Or shall I say, yet another dream come true.

It's the rich life that matters, rich with your kids, rich with your partner, rich with your friends, rich with the impact you want to have on this planet, rich in terms of successful business, where you feel a sense of meaning and enjoyment, all of these things, they are so much more valuable than living a balanced and boring life.

Balanced life never worked for me, I do everything 110% and I would be tortured by balance.

Try and see how it goes for you. Just enjoy everything and every moment to its absolute fullest. I assure you, you'll never go back to the bore of balance.

Be where you are right now.

When it comes to my health I simply picked what works the best for me. I saw fast results with Keto and I was able to sustain it. I got so passionate about it. I devoted a good portion of this book toward sharing it with you all. **Spoiler alert: more books like this are already in the works** ☺.

What I am trying to tell you is that being where you are is totally ok. Be unapologetic. Live on your own terms; take as much time as you need to figure out what those terms are and what it is that you want, and don't waste energy concerning yourself with what others think. You are not living for others but for you. Who cares what others think? I know I don't. This doesn't mean I don't take others well being into consideration. I am sure you understand what I mean by when I say, do you, live for you.

I realize I say "I don't care" a lot … and I mean a lot. With the eye roll, if you know what I mean.

When I say that I don't care though, what I mean is this, nothing is going to stop me, and nothing will take my momentum away. I know where I am going. I also know that not everyone has my vision and that's totally ok. We are all here for our own purpose, and knowing what your purpose is winning half of the battle. The other half is just sticking to it, like your life depends on it, be consistent with it, be stubborn about it and don't give up. You planted a seed. You already know your end result. It's already done. The seed doesn't bloom the day you planted it. It, like us, has its own time, so be patient and don't doubt yourself on your journey to your own greatness.

Never, not ever, will I modify myself to please others or try to make them feel ok by adjusting my own level of consciousness to match that of theirs. Luckily, I don't have people like that around me today. I love feeling alive, everything I do in my life is making me feel alive, and that's due to my ability to make decisions without hesitating anymore. By just following my heart and not ignoring my hunches. Thanks to YAGE.

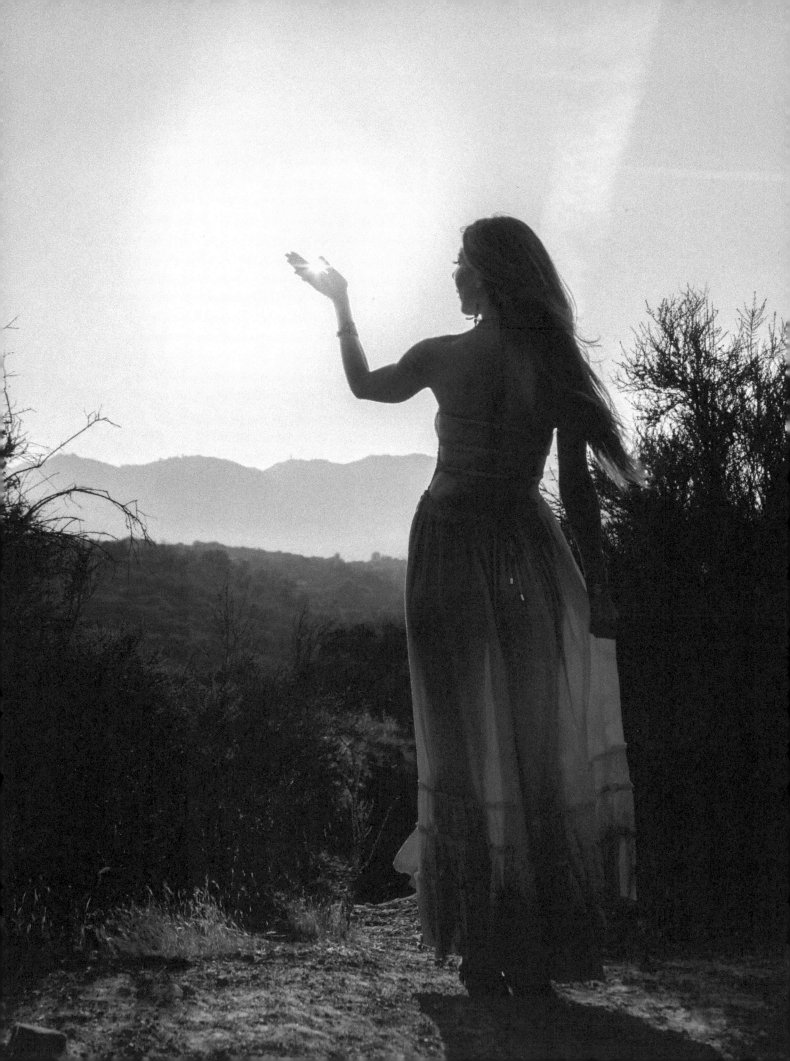

My heart is my guide and I am on purpose.

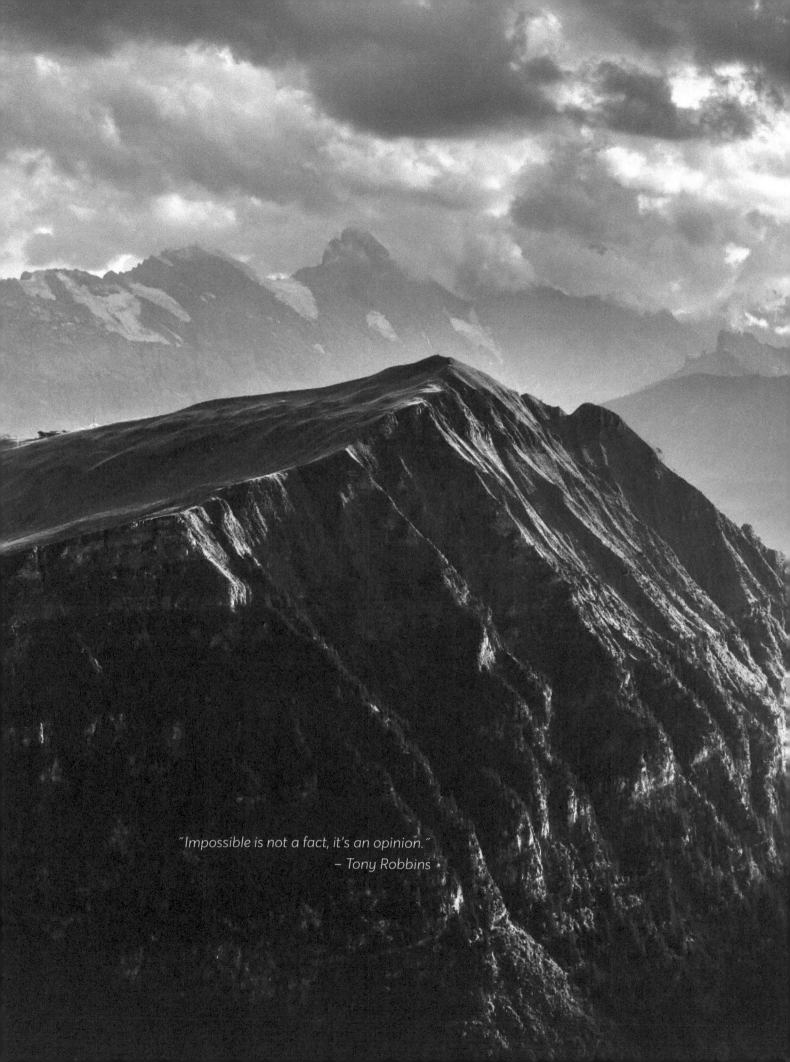

"Impossible is not a fact, it's an opinion."
– Tony Robbins

BREATHE INTO YOUR HEART

The heart-centered life. Close your eyes and take a deep breath in, yes now, take a deep breath, see your heart in your mind, breathe into it, see it's beating, see the color … now breathe out.

You can also put your hand on your heart, breathe in and out, feel your heart. Visualize the energy moving through it. The energy is light, yes; visualize this energy as being white light, circulating, pulsating, reverberating, *resonating* with each breath. Do this as many times during the day as possible. You will feel so grateful to be alive. Just like they say, if you want to experience a miracle, take a breath. Amen to that.

The heart is this amazing machine that keeps us going, gives us life.
Think about your heart as the energy center, like a car battery. All energy is created from it. It makes our blood circulate, it keeps us alive. If you are not aware of your thoughts, meaning if you don't have the leash on your mind, and just let it wander around, and allow it to do whatever it thinks, then you are in trouble. Controlling your thoughts is the first thing on your to do list. Meaning, when you start to be aware of your thoughts, you can control where the energy is flowing, therefore the feeling is created.

If you want to have a beautiful life and if you don't want to live in default mode then you need to be aware of your thoughts. Listen to them. What are they saying? Is your mind in the future? Or is it in the past? Do you spend your days thinking about what happened, or what will happen, instead of staying in the present moment?

Your thoughts have power to change how you feel, and how you feel will change your outcome in life. Your heart will react to your thoughts the minute the thoughts travel to your heart. You will start to feel everything. How you feel is a great indicator of the energy you are emanating. If you are not ok or feeling half assed, like something is off, then that means something is off, therefore immediately change your focus.

What we think about is so important that it shapes our 3D reality. You always have a choice to be happy or miserable. Right now, as I am writing these pages, I am going through a heartache myself, it's not always easy to remember what I preach as I hit roadblocks of my own. Because when you are hurting, you don't remember anything you know, mental shut down. The pain takes over. This is why pain is the greatest teacher of all. Because of this, most people will be scared to face healing. This is also another reason so many people are on medication to numb their feelings. It is not a walk in the park. Dealing with your dark side is a warrior's feat. I just made a decision to deal with it once and for all rather than living in the same old experiences. That only perpetuates the cycle of more pain.

I am a warrior. I can do it and because I made that decision, I CAN. I am now more aware of my thoughts because I have learned to know better.

Now, I see everything as, it's happening for me, not to me. I am protected and loved by the source, the spirit, the God, whatever you want to name it. There is this universal love that doesn't judge. We all have to go through lessons so we can learn so that we can remember who we really are.

Lessons hurt, but in order for us to grow we need them. The good part is that today my recovery is faster, unlike before where I would stay in bed for days, not seeing or talking to anyone.

As I continue to learn to breathe into my heart and to let go, I release blockages faster and easier. When there is a blockage, your heart will hurt, your energy will be low, and you won't feel like doing anything. With blockages, you will feel depressed, not want to get out of bed, you'll hide, feeling hopeless and powerless. Yes, I know, I have been through it all.

Feeling rejected, or as though you're not enough will cut your life source energy. When I feel sad, I usually try to sit in the quiet and listen to my inner talk. It's like there is someone else who lives there. I call her "she" because sometimes I can't believe I am thinking those things. I feel it's so much easier to be negative then be positive and optimistic. I am sure you can relate.

She never shuts up, she is mean at times, I watch her. I don't fall into her traps anymore, the mind games, but if I wasn't aware of my inner voice, she (I mean my ego self) would keep me bitter or sad or feeling like shit even longer. And I remember, I don't like feeling shitty.

Now I see my inner talk, I consciously make a decision to create better thoughts. It's ok to feel the pain. When the pain is moving through your heart it will hurt, but it will hurt for a second or a day or two. Not like before, years and years of remembering and reliving it. You have to work with the pain. It's trying to teach you something so you won't repeat it again. You can't suppress it. You can't hide behind a mask and pretend all is well when you know all is not well.

Take your time to be alone, cry it out if you have to. Deal with it head on. Otherwise, it will always resurface. You can be sure of that. It will shape your future reality, because you will close your heart and, when your heart is closed, the life force doesn't pass through. You will be so scared to live fully just to avoid feeling pain again, you won't let anyone get close to you and you will build walls, you will be on guard, you will shut down, and that's just not the way we are supposed to live. We are here in this human form as a soul to experience joy and love so we can ascend.

Don't let one bad experience, or even several bad experiences ruin your life. Of course it hurts, it hurts like MF. I am going through it right now, but I also know I honor this pain, I see it as a gift. My pain is trying to teach me something so I won't ever have to feel this way again. It may be the best gift ever, allowing me to breathe and let it go, and giving me the knowledge that I will heal from it. I know if you let this pass through, you will have a healed heart. The energy needs to flow. Remember the heart is the white light and the battery for life, we need it for everything, and everything in life depends on it.

I see the pain, I accept the pain, and with each breath I say, let it go, and I literally see the pain leaving my heart. I repeat this until I feel better. I keep telling myself, this is just an experience. LET IT GO.

Always remember, obstacles will make you stronger, and also remember, right now, as you are breathing, it's the only thing that matters. Time doesn't exist; the past and the future are only in your memory and imagination. You live what you think about, you can't change the past. What's done is done, we can never go back and fix it, and no one gets a second chance. You learned, you moved on, no more pity party. You are here now reading this book. You are here now. All you have is your breath. Focus on it now, the couch you are sitting on, the room you are in, the sounds you are hearing.

As you get what you think about, why would you want to keep thinking about what happened yesterday unless you want to create the same experience? Use your imagination, create your tomorrow, we have that power within us. We are creators. Allow yourself to move through your pain, grieve, cry, scream, but don't hold onto it, the more you hold onto it, the longer you will keep creating the same experiences. Who wants that? I am done with that. You are done with that. We are done with that.

The past does not equal the future.

LETTING GO

Ahhhhhhhh, deep breath, this is the ultimate challenge. It seems so hard to do. I personally know this very well, because I used to get stuck in stories of the past.

When I get into my head I like taking long walks to clear it. I usually go to Zuma in Malibu. It's my favorite beach in California, because it's long and beautiful. You can really get into a meditative space. You walk, and walk, and walk and the beach still keeps going. On these walks I tend to listen to my own inner talk and I watch everything, I see and hear every thought with so much focus and attention.

On one of these particular walks, I was dealing with heartache; it has been a crazy roller coaster of two years of drama with this guy that I really have a connection with. I can't explain it. It was like an addiction and I finally had the courage to walk away. Which I have tried to do in the past maybe twenty times, maybe more, and I had failed every time.

After the days would go by, I would get worse instead of getting better. I would keep thinking about all of our beautiful days together, to ease the pain, facing pain is not easy. I would rather stay in memories and think of our beautiful days so it would not hurt, I would think about our secret meet ups, fun times and I would keep torturing myself.

I was not aware of it back then as I am today. I was just reflecting my pain to the universe, and that's what I was getting back multiplied. You only get what you are. You never get what you want. I could not get my mind just to stop it, stop it all together, I knew he was bad for me, but I don't mean he is a bad person, what I mean is that really, he was bad for me and I could not get my head to stop thinking about us, him. I was not breathing, my chest would hurt when I took a breath in, my heart would feel like a rock because it would hurt so bad.

I knew my heart was closed up, and I also knew the heart was the energy center, so basically, I have been paralyzing myself for the past two years with this back and forth and heartache. I have never felt so insignificant. My heart was so congested.

A congested heart is not a healthy heart. If your heart is not working properly, nothing in your life will work properly. By now I knew this very well and when I say nothing, it includes your work life as well. The energy is produced in the heart. It's like having a super fast car but you don't have gas so you can't drive the car. What's the point in having a fast car if you are going to keep it in the garage all the time? It's the same thing. It's such a waste of beautiful, powerful energy. Remember we never get back this moment ever again.

The urge to leave this guy came to my heart a long time ago, but I entirely ignored the hunch, the gut feeling, because I was addicted to him.

I really loved him, loved him unconditionally, I still do, and probably always will. But this didn't mean I had to stay in an unhealthy relationship. I was so aware of everything, and knew deep down in my gut I had to let it (him) go.

As I was walking that day on Zuma, I was listening to my inner talk, the girl who lives there said, 'you are used to this pain.' I nodded my head, and I caught myself agreeing with her, OMG yes, I have been here before, I had this pain before, I've had it actually three times, I have only fallen in love three times.

Wow, that's a hard pill to swallow, so I asked my inner voice, where did I go wrong? She said, look at how all of them started, then I went all the way back to the beginning of each relationship and they had one thing in common.

They all showed me a major red flag within three months and I ignored it every time.

I settled, I thought if I loved them so much then they would love me the way I was expecting to be loved and they will never hurt me again. Well, they all tried, but they all failed. Oh yes, you guessed it, I stayed anyway.

First realization, I ignored my hunch, I did not honor myself, I settled. I accepted the fact that they did something to hurt me and I did not do anything about it. This gave them the impression that I was okay with the way they treated me. I take accountability for my part now. I moved forward and I'm stronger now, but back then I believed that it was my fault. That was normal to me. I was used to being that way.

But in the meantime, I kept eating myself up, I was losing pieces of myself, losing self-respect, feeling insecure and feeling not enough.

Why did I do that? Why did I stay? I didn't know. I didn't feel I was loveable at all.

My father left my mother when I was two years old. Both my sister and I believed that we did not matter. We were both products of an environment that we could not control. We had programmed beliefs, behaviors and understandings. It started at a very young age. I did not understand the concept back then because I normalized it within me.

So up until this last experience, I had no freaking clue. In this last experience, when I had my heart diced into little nothings, I realized that I was responsible for all.

They didn't promise me the world and took it back. I settled. I settled for the breadcrumbs and that's exactly what I was getting in return. This time I was not satisfied with the breadcrumbs. My inner voice has been talking to me   probably all my life, but since I was so clogged up with old beliefs and I had never listened to my hunches before, in fact I don't think I even noticed them before. Until it got louder and louder, and the pain got bigger and bigger. I was not able to breathe anymore. The change had to come and it had to come now. I could no longer live this way.

Oh my, and all that was my fault, I was responsible for it. What a relief. Now I had the power to fix it. I'd blamed the world before. No more blame game, no more giving power away. It was me who was going to do something about it.

Manipulating love, I would give and give and give, so in return I deserved to be loved, that was my game plan and if they didn't behave, I assumed they would feel bad, and act better. Oh boy...

Up until I asked myself the big question. Why did I settle knowing that I deserved better? I had no idea what I was doing wrong. That was my pattern. Since that was my pattern, and since I had no clue where it was coming from, I kept creating the same relationship with different faces.

I have done so much work on myself, I know YAGE was trying to show me this as well in many of my ceremonies, but I even ignored her.

Now I know what I am doing. Now I am conscious of it and I know how to fix it. I had no clue before, but when I finally understood, I needed to talk to Taita. I needed to drink Yage and we needed to organize this. We had to clear the congestion of my energy center. My lovely, big heart needed my help.

Congestion creates disease and an unhappy, unsatisfied life. I needed circulation, I needed energy flow, and I needed my heart to beat again. I needed my heart to belong to me again and not to my past memories.

I had a day of silence. I took a day off. I stayed in my room. I was sitting on my bed, thinking, *how did I get here?* I was sad, I started to pray … and I asked, *what do I do? Please help me figure this out … Please give me a sign.*

As I was sitting and watching the walls, something on my bookshelf, where I have a massive collection of metaphysical books, caught my eye. I got to my feet, I stood in front of it, and I picked up a book by Michael A. Singer, titled, *The Untethered Soul.*

I started reading it. I had read this book a long time ago, as I have read many books like it before as well, but now I revisit them for no particular reason, aside from knowing that I have a different perspective than I did when I first read them years ago. I have changed a lot but I still love my same old books. Books are medicine. You will find exactly what you need when you need it. They speak to you, they tell you exactly what you need to hear to move on, grow and learn. I love books.

As I was reading Singer's book again I realized that I was given a solution. The author was talking about the heart and how to clear the congestion of past traumas. Bingo, jackpot. This was exactly the medicine I needed. I read the entire book in one sitting. I was sick of the same old patterns. I was determined to fix my heart.

He said, sit in silence, breathe into your heart and breathe out and mentally think, LET IT GO.

I was like, is that it? I was so confused that it was so easy. It can't be that easy. I read it again and again, breathe into your heart, breathe out, and say **let it go.**

I said ok, tomorrow I am going to go for my walk, I am going to breathe into my heart, breathe out, and say **let it go.**

The next day, I went to Zuma, my favorite long and beautiful beach that I mentioned before. I walked and I started to look for a place where there was no one, I felt like being alone. I also wanted to sit on the sand; I wanted to be connected to the mother earth.

It was such a beautiful day, perfect breeze on my face, the sun wasn't too hot, I felt everything on my skin, and I was in the present moment. No one was around me and I had found the best spot. I sat there, I had music with me, and I used a heart opener sound bath. Anything at 528hz will do.

Subconscious is often impressed through the music. Music has a 4D quality and releases the soul from imprisonment, it makes things possible and easy to accomplish. Music releases the imagination and it induces the imagination. This is one of the best tools you have to meditate.

So, ready, set, go!

I sat, I took a couple deep slow breaths in and out, and before I closed my eyes, I looked out at the ocean, it was massive, endless, and I suddenly realized I was part of that. I felt one with it and I went into the spirit world.

I continued to take deep breaths, in and out, and as I was breathing, I was visualizing my heart, after about 5 minutes or so, I got really into it, thoughts were coming in and out, I just kept going back to visualizing my heart, I was staring at it, it was huge, and it was black.

I was not breathing deeply because it would hurt. It would literally, viscerally… hurt to breathe in… hurt to breathe out, my ribs would physically, unbearably hurt.

So, I asked quietly in my mind, where is the pain? I never stopped breathing into it, I kept breathing through it, and it was all the way on the bottom back part of my heart. I saw it, it was all black.

Then something magical happened, I saw Taita, and three fairy kind of looking spirits, they were dancing around me, one of them started to work on my heart, one of them was washing me with the ocean water as I was breathing, the other one was taking my breath into my dark heart. Then my heart started turning pink, from the bottom and traveling upward to the top, I just kept breathing. I saw my heart was changing color, I saw it, it was a miracle, the entire black part almost only at the top, I just kept breathing into the pain, and kept saying, let it go, Julyet, let it go, I just kept repeating it as I was watching my heart turning into pink again.

And it disappeared, it went into my throat, I felt it in my throat then the energy moved up and released through my tears. I started crying, I was healed, I was healed, I took a massive breath in and I didn't hurt, I got my heart back. OMG I was crying now with joy, I felt the tears coming down my cheeks.

I lost all resentment toward my exes, toward my dad as well. I felt no pain. I felt free. There was this massive empty space where I could take a huge breath in, the pain transmuted into peace. I didn't realize the pain had been taking up so much space in my heart. I felt emptied of it. Almost didn't even remember what it felt like before. All I had to do was make a decision, make a decision to let go and move on. We all have a choice. What is meant for me will be mine. But the beliefs I had been holding onto wouldn't allow me to surrender. I was creating from memories not from the present moment, never again.

Now, it's a new playing field. If it's already done, if I have created my life, and believe, and it's already done the way I want it to be, then I have no reason to question my creation. That is my new affirmation, when I feel doubt creeping up; I keep going back to, IT IS DONE. It's done, it's done, and it's done. This will only work once you accept the present moment and become absolutely ok with it.

I would like to paraphrase a quote from SADHGURU here. This is one of the best teachings I have come across.
"Living for the moment is for the pleasure seeker's life. Living in the moment is not something you invented. Life is always in the moment. If you are aware of that you will live a balanced and sensible life. If you are unaware of it, you will get into hellish states and foolish things in life."

So living in the moment is not something that you have to tell yourself. I must live in the moment.

Whatever is happening with you, whatever the emotion, whatever the thought, whatever the experience, simply seeing that this moment is inevitable the way it is.

When you do that the next moment is a new possibility. Only if you accept this moment absolutely the way it is, the next moment becomes a new possibility.

Otherwise you will drag the past into the future.

You are talking about the future but you really do not know anything about the future.

Your mind only knows the past. What you call the future is that you take a piece of the past and apply make-up on it and you think it's the future. Improved past is what you call the future.

Dragging your past into the future is a sure way of destroying your life. It is a sure way of ruling out all new possibilities.

So if you are not accepting the inevitability of what is there right now naturally your past will extend into your future. Future will not be a new possibility; it will be a repetition of the past. Do you see the cycle of nonsense happening again and again in your life?

This is because you are not accepting the current moment as it is; therefore you are dragging the past into the future.

It is not your fate. It is not God's will. It is you.

If you are accepting everything the way it is, you say, my responsibility is limitless, you have accepted everything the way it is."

Thank you Sadguru.

I am free at last.

Now, I sit in heart meditation everyday. I made a new habit. Now, I choose the time according to my own freedom and my own free will, I don't have a set time for it. I don't like rules much, in case that hasn't become obvious by now! So, when I say find what works for you, I really mean that from the bottom of my heart. Let it go, release your heart from the darkness, set your heart free.

Otherwise, you will stay in darkness. Until you learn how to see in darkness.
Now I have newfound self-respect, I don't skip any of my hunches, they are my protectors, my guides. I will not downplay my feelings anymore.

I am loveable and I am more than enough, I am love.

If you are going to settle, settle with your soul. Trust it, surrender to it. It will never fail you.

Take ownership, don't give anyone else responsibility for your happiness or for your unhappiness, you are the creator, you are making the decisions, you are doing it, it has nothing to do with anyone but you.

Get your power back; life will flourish in front of your eyes. I am living proof. Try it. You have nothing to lose but yourself. Don't carry your past into your future, accept what it is fully now. Take time to be in silence so you can hear. I love you with all my heart.

And now say it out loud ALL IS WELL.

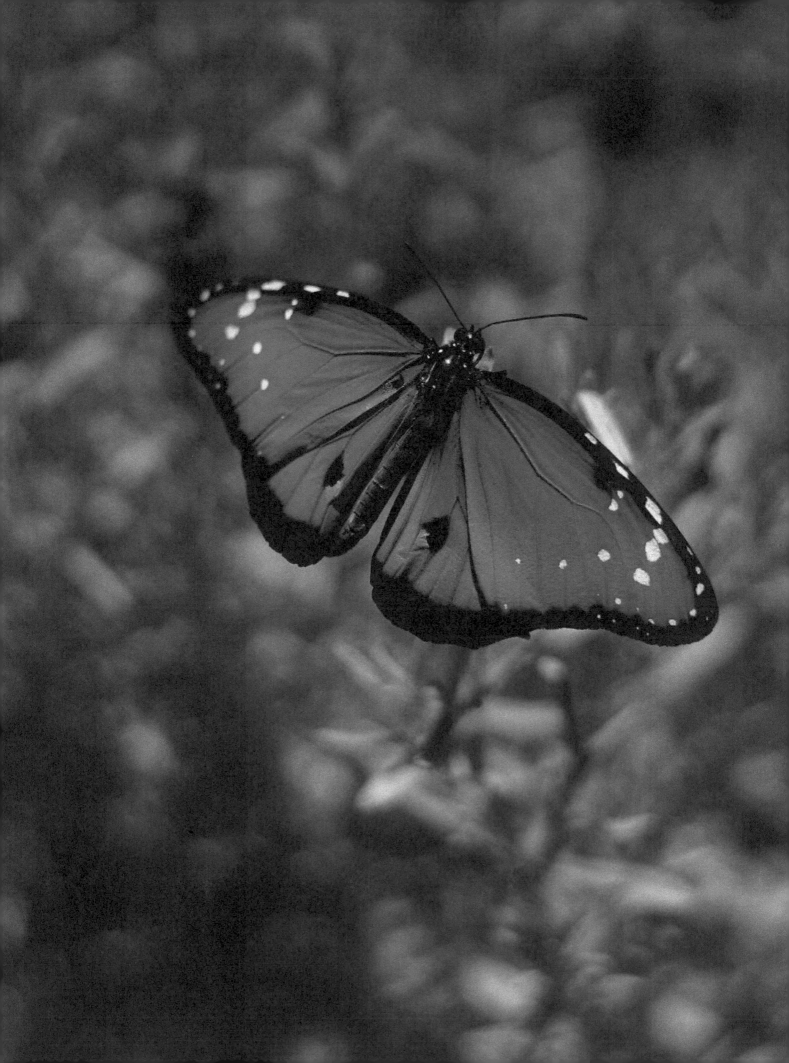

All is well.

CHAPTER 3

CREATION PROCESS

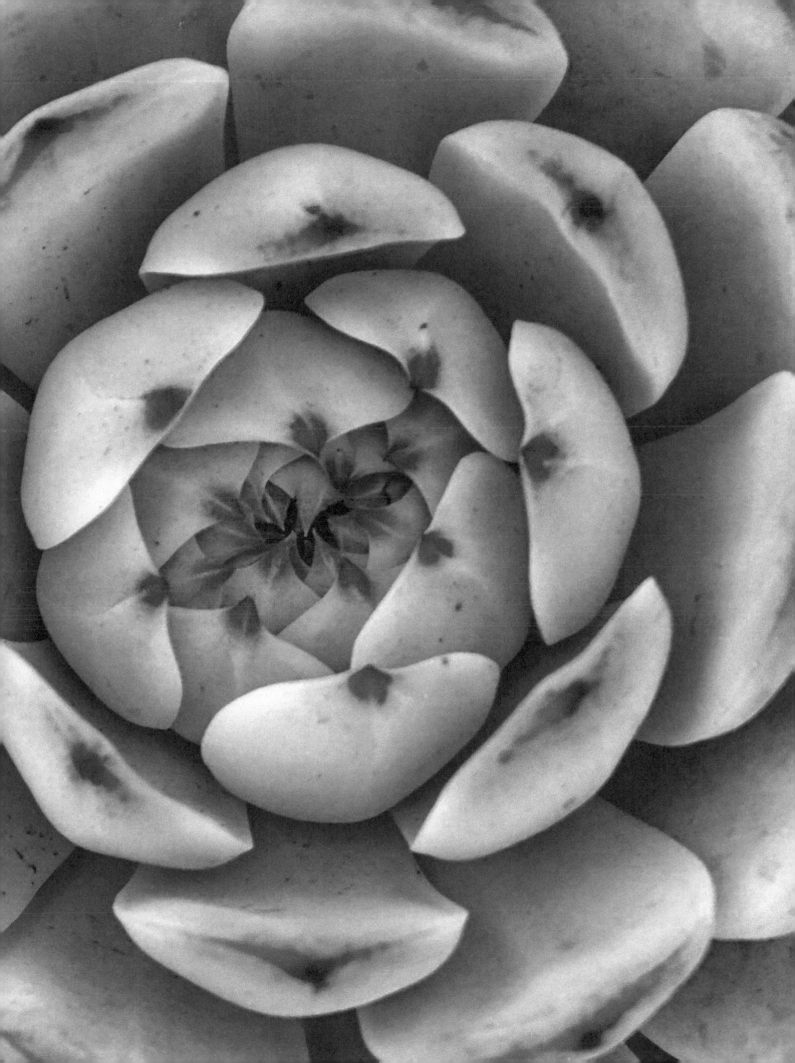

CREATION PROCESS

This is the fun part. How do we create anything out of thin air? So far the life you are living is the one you believed you could have, you probably created it on default according to the way you were raised. Your current beliefs have a major part in it.

We only live the life that we believe we can have. So, now you know that you have created what you have so far, you now also know that you can always change it.

Design it the way you desire it. Before we get started, I want you to ask yourself. What do I want? Think about that, as if you have no limitations, think of what you want, really, dive in. Close your eyes and imagine, where would you want to be? What does your home look like, what kind of relationships do you have? How much money do you have? What kind of job do you have? What do you look like? Are you in the best shape ever? How would it feel to have all your desires come true?

The universe only gives you what you are, not what you want. It will always reflect back, like a mirror. Think of it as if you are looking into the mirror, if you smile it smiles back, if you frown, it will frown back.

If you are feeling shitty, you will get back shitty. In order to create anything, the first thing you need to do is check to see how you are feeling. Are you feeling excited or desperate?

If you are not feeling well, then your first task is to change your state of mind, and you can do this by changing focus. For example, let's say, your boyfriend didn't call you, and now you are really pissed, thinking all sorts of bad things, and now you are getting angrier by the minute. When you notice you are building anger, immediately, change your focus, play music, jump up and down, watch a funny cat video, call your friend, (don't call her/him to complain about him) talk about random things, work out, go for a walk, do anything to change your negative state. I usually listen to Neville Goddard. I learned so much from him. He is one of my favorite teachers.

If you are feeling upset and for some reason you can't change your state, then sit with it, give yourself permission to feel the pain, feel it, breathe into it, cry if it makes you feel better, but know that you are not going to stay there for a long time. You are just allowing it to move through you. In this case, I usually go for long walks and listen to medicine music (my favorite medicine music artist is JUAN DAVID

MUNOZ FERNANDEZ, you can find him on iTunes or juanda.hearnow.com) and I breathe into my heart. I just focus on breathing in and out of my heart. This will move the energy. You just try to stay in the present moment.

After you feel better you can start creating. Remember, you don't want to stay in a shitty mood for too long. Otherwise it will become your personality, and no one likes a shitty person! You will lose people around you, also remember, no one cares, in this mood, you will only hurt yourself. Stop it now. Move on.

Understanding what you don't want is a great way to find out what you do want. Beat the drum of what you want. The more you talk about what you want is a great way to change your mood. You will feel excited about everything and you will mirror that to the universe.

Since the universe acts as a mirror, we have to be careful not to stay in the past, or live in the future, what I mean is that if you stay in the past, you will only reflect those feelings, therefore you will relive the past over and over, until you understand that you are actually creating your life by how you feel. Nothing will change in your life until you understand this.

And if you are dreaming of the future or thinking and saying, I am going to be rich, or I will be married, or I will get the job then will always stay in the wanting stage but never arriving at your destination. You are a watcher from a distance; you are not acting like it's already done. You have to see yourself at the next stage, which is after your wishes are done, what will you be doing? See and feel yourself in it. BE IT. You wouldn't say, ahhh, when I am rich, or ahhh, when I get married. Since you already are rich and married or whatever the desire you want to experience is in your possession, you would be talking about, where would you be going for vacation with your husband or wife, or you would be talking about where you will be investing the money you already have. That's a totally different vibration, it doesn't come from lack, therefore you are reflecting to the universe you are not in lack, on the contrary, you are full in everything. And this way, your only outcome will be to get back even more full in life on every aspect of it.

Dr. Joe Dispenza explains it well, he says; this is the time in history is not enough to know but this is the time in history to know how. When you unify with your heart, you go from someone to no one to everyone. Surrender and get out of the way. Heart is the center of oneness, center of wholeness, your first step to divinity, your bridge. Your connection to the unified field.

Now, this is what I learned from Dr. Joe Dispenza on creating what I want. This is a simple meditation, which you can do anytime.

Step 1. Turn all the electronics off, no cell, no tv, power down your computer. Sit your body down and close your eyes.

Step 2. Take some breaths to center yourself. When you center attention into the present moment, you will have more energy to create with. When your mind wanders to the predictable future or the familiar past, that's normal. Just become aware of it and keep working on settling yourself back into the present moment, I usually do that by breathing into my heart, I visualize my heart beating.

Step 3. Ask yourself, what do I want in my life? Take time to answer this question, the answer will come to you, just get present, focus on your heart, your heart will always speak to you, you just have to get in your mind to hear it. As you begin contemplating, you are changing your brain. When you start getting your answers notice how that makes you feel.

Step 4. Once you catch the feeling, stay there. And see what you would be doing if you were to realize your wishes, if you were asking for the love of your life, and now you have it, how would you feel? How would you behave? What will you be doing with him? Marinate in this feeling. Juice it. Remember to go to the next stage of having it.

Step 5. Decide what thoughts you want to bring to your future. Write them down, decide what emotions no longer belong to your future, this means if you want to be wealthy, you can't bring any "lack" with you. If you want to be healthy, you can't take fear with you.

You have to act and feel as if it's already done. If it's already done, you are no longer asking for the money or the love or the health. It's done.

You have to have the confidence in your creation that it's already **DONE.**

Have I said that enough?
It is done, it is done, it is done, it is done, and it is done.

You have to be one with your desired outcome. You can't talk about it as if it will happen in the near future. You have to go beyond that. You have to go to the next stage of after having what you desire, what would you be doing?

This makes it more concrete now that it's already been done. Now celebrate it. If you were to ask for a promotion, and you got it, what would follow the promotion? Can you see yourself with your friends? Are they throwing a party to congratulate you? Visualize it, you are in there with them, seeing their faces, hearing their words to you. Telling you how happy they are for you.

Stay in that feeling, and when for whatever reason, the old feelings come up, say it out loud, "nope I am not going there, my wishes are already done!"

I bet you have a smile on your face right now, because I do. I have nothing to worry about. Remember, it is done, it is done, and it is done. Do this in your Imagination before you fall asleep. When you go to bed, see everything in your mind. I do this every night, I swear, I fall asleep with a smile on my face. Let your subconscious marinate in what you created, and believe that it will come on it's own time, whatever you are creating will be your physical reality. You planted a seed; now believe that it's yours. It is already done.

You planted a seed into your subconscious, it is like being pregnant, there is no such thing as being a little bit pregnant, the seed is going to grow, and give birth. It's as simple and as concrete as that. You just have to believe and feel that it's already done. Every imaginative act will rise into a fact. That is the law of the universe.

It's done.

CHAPTER 4

WHAT IS KETO

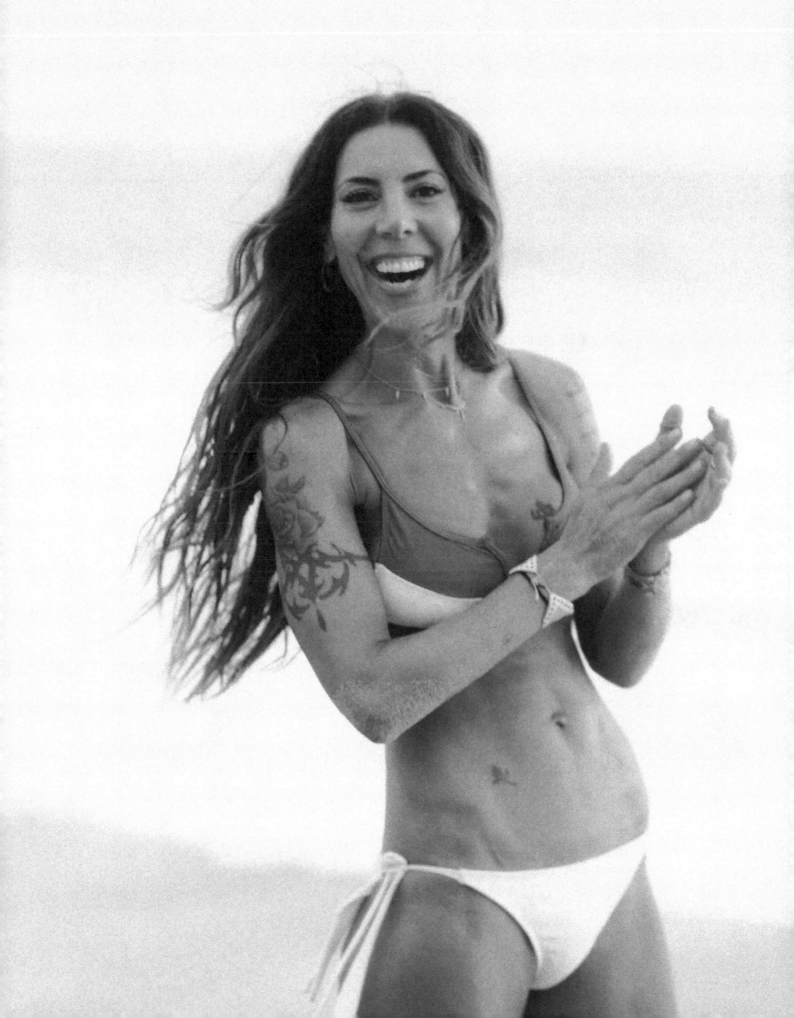

WHAT IS KETO?

Keto is a metabolic state of ketosis. Your body burns fat as a fuel instead of insulin (sugar). Keto is high in natural nutritious fats, moderate in protein, ultra-low in carbohydrates.

What Is The Difference Between Keto And Paleo?

The ketogenic diet is focused on manipulating the three macronutrients, which are fat, protein, and carbs. The Paleo diet is more about eliminating dairy and grains and processed foods.

I like both, but keto works better for me. Try both and what agrees with you, there is no one way fits all.

How Did I Start My Keto Journey?

Well, it's a bit of a long story but I guess that's why I'm writing a book about it☺.

Everything started with this pandemic, and I do believe that one day we'll look back and thank God for it.

I was in panic mode and super stressed, until I learned to surrender to it. I was just home, with my kids, watching tons of Netflix, reading, cleaning the house, organizing drawers, I started fixing things that had needed my attention for so long, things I never made time for before. In the meantime, I started to cook a lot of food out of boredom. I never really had a big appetite but I was cooking anyway, piling food in the fridge. I was eating as I pleased, and not moving much, the gyms were closed, I didn't feel motivated at all and I was falling into the monotony of lock down living … But cool side note, I probably finished Netflix☺.

One day, I wanted to watch the Matrix. This was maybe my 6th time seeing the movie since it was released 6 years ago. I was watching it with a new eye, with a new consciousness. Haha, before Yage, after Yage ☺.

So that night I went to bed and in my dream I took the red pill. I went where Neo went, and there I was told, in order for me to get where I want to go, I need to detox, and clean my body. The whole experience was so real to me, I couldn't believe it. I literally, well, literally in my dream, took the red pill.

The next day, I decided to do a water fast. I just knew that's what I needed to do to start. I was so determined to follow the instructions, and I did, and the rest is a history ☺.

I failed many times until I was able to do ten days. After that, I was a whole new Julyet; there was no way I was going back to eating wheat or sugar.

I felt brand new, clear minded, and full of energy and motivation. My skin looked amazing, I was in great shape and I just started to appreciate and love my body even more. You can't fix the body you don't love.

I love my body, I want to take care of it and now, I've upgraded to a Ferrari whereas before I was maybe a Jeep… (I drive a Jeep and I love my Jeep - but you know what I mean).

When you reach the full potential of your body and see what it can do for you, you will never want to mess with that, you want to make sure it is well taken care of.

When you are no longer controlled by hunger, you are finally ready to get in the driver seat, and get behind your own wheel (I promise, you're going to love being a new Ferrari!). You are now in control of when you stop and when you go, you, not your haywire hunger. Decide when to eat, what to eat and when you've had enough.

Keto is another factor that literally changed everything for me. I am so passionate about it. That's why I wanted to share all of it. Now I am down to one meal a day, and that one meal is the perfect meal. I love food shopping. I love preparing my food. I have so much appreciation for farmers, for the stores, for the drivers who deliver our food to our door steps, I can't wait to grow my own food, that is on my bucket list.

Ever since I started paying more attention to what I am putting into my body, I started to shop more mindfully, I want to know about what I'm putting into this body I have come to love and treasure so much. I want to learn how my veggies are grown and what kind of soil quality the farmer is using. Everything you eat becomes a part of you, becomes you. This information may sound a bit crazy to you as you read it for the first time but I promise, by the time you finish this book, you'll see it as a simple fact and be baffled at how it didn't make sense to you before.

Let's talk about FAT

Let's talk about the right fats. Why is it so important to get the right fat on Keto when you can still lose weight eating even the wrong fats? In Ketosis, the body uses fat as fuel, so regardless you will lose weight but you will hit a plateau.

Yes, maybe you lost a bunch of fat, but now you are inflamed, which is not healthy at all, inflammation can cause a myriad of diseases.

To live longer and to lose weight, ketosis is massively important, when you know what to do, ketosis is the best tool to craft your body, and your health. Like an artist, you can create anything once you have the right tools.

Fats you eat are either going to be used for energy (jet fuel), or building blocks. As a building block do you know what percentage of your body is a starch (which very simply explained is also a carbohydrate)?

Less than 1%. So you don't need carbs as building blocks, you need fat. 45% of your cell membrane is fat, saturated fat and your brain needs fat.

Now you have to look at what kind of fats you are consuming?

The best building block for fat is saturated fat, that's a foundational fat, saturated fats are awesome, because they don't oxidize and they don't break easily, and they are stable.

The white fat that surrounds your organs or that is under your skin is the most flexible. If you eat something that contains omega 6, it will store in the white fat cells. Oxidize omega 6 is very common, what you are going to get is more white fat cells from it, and all these white fat cells mostly causing the inflammation.

This is why people often fail when first attempting the Keto Diet, because they are thinking all fats are equal, they didn't eat any carbs, just had fried food. Well, guess what? You can't eat fried foods.

If you are eating a lot of fat, you need to eat clean, undamaged fat.

Basically it's not just the type of fat you are consuming, but how the fat has been treated. Yes you heard me. That actually matters.

The difference between fat and carbs is that carbs are only a source of fuel (cheap fuel) where fat is a ("jet fuel") fat is a building block. So you don't want to oxidize fat in your system, it will slow you down, and get you sick.

You want to make sure your fat source is clean. Saturated fat is the best choice. You don't want to over cook your fat, but use high heat tolerance oils when cooking, (avocado oil is my favorite, my favorite brand is Primal Kitchen) never cook with olive oil, it gets rancid.

Staying In Ketosis All The Time Is Not Healthy

You may end up with keto flu, or sleepless nights. Your body needs insulin as well, small amounts, especially for the ladies around your moon cycle.

Introducing insulin about four or five days before your moon cycle is important for your T4-T3 conversion, and you need insulin for that. Once you get your moon, you can go back to fasting or ketosis again. When I say insulin, I don't mean go devour a whole pizza, or bread, although I recommend healthy versions of it, sprouted sourdough is my choice. There are also other types of healthy carbs and fruits that you can introduce to your diet at this time. I go for fruits that I usually don't eat when I'm fasting or when I'm in ketosis. My favorite is watermelon, I love frozen blueberries, any kind of berries are my picks, I also do sweet potato, I love white rice, you will be saying, oh but that's not keto, well, I'm always going to eat what I want to eat, I don't really listen to many strict advices, because if my body wants it, I will go for it. I have self-control. I love myself, I do know my limits, but if I want a bit of white rice, I will damn well eat white rice! I usually go for sushi this time of the month. It is my responsibility to know what my limits are, I love taking care of my health and therefore I will never cheat.

As a child, I grew up on stage, I was a ballerina, I remember my coach used to say, everyday when you get to that stage you owe it to the people who came to see you to give your best, whoever is watching you may be seeing you for the first time, you can not half ass it, if you want to be the best, you have to give your best all the time. You are as good as your last show. What kind of impression do you want to leave, when you go to bed at night, can you honestly tell yourself you gave it all? Can you? If the answer is yes, it's amazing, if the answer is no, then you aim for the best version the next day.

Fitness On Keto

I have not been doing intense workouts since starting keto. Ever since my gym was closed due to Covid-19 pandemic. I was just doing my home workouts and long walks, I have lost 15lbs.

I lift weights three times a week, leg day, abs day, arms and back day. Back to legs day and repeat the processes with two days off in between.
The other days, I still do my long walks. I am not a big fan of cardio, but I am keeping myself busy and keeping my heartbeat up, which helps burn fat faster.
I usually do all my workouts in a fasted state, so I'm making sure that my body is using fat as a source of energy (jet fuel)☺.

Also, I make sure to take my morning cocktail with salt, lemon and cream of tartar (potassium) definitely before my workout (see recipe chapter), this will help with electrolytes while you are working out in a fasted stage, so you won't get dizzy, or feel weak.

With your morning cocktail, make sure to also take your vitamin D, and at night before bed take your magnesium. Since we don't eat standard carbs, our bodies don't retain water (this is why we don't look or feel bloated because we're not!) but, losing electrolytes is unhealthy and will make you feel weak and hungry. Don't fall for it. It's a quick fix.

Right now, I am on the maintenance level; therefore I am really not pushing myself as hard as I would if I were in the weight loss stage. I am now excited to be shaping my body the way I want it to look. I feel I have a blank canvas.

But if you are trying to lose weight, it's a great idea to utilize cardio at least 3-4 times a week, do whatever you like doing and sleep really well. Weight loss happens while you are sleeping which is also when your muscles heal most properly.

I still do my 18/6 five days a week, I still do 24 hours of fasting one day a week and that day I don't work out. It's also my quiet day. I rest and meditate and do inner work. Lastly, one day a week, I do keto flex, meaning, I eat three meals a day and I don't go into ketosis.

Once you get the hang of it, you will see how easy this will be for you, now you are in charge of everything. You are driving your Ferrari. This is the best feeling ever. Your weight is not controlling you anymore, you control everything. You've reached the epitome of what it means to be free.

Sleep

Sleep is one of the most important parts of your health and your well-being. When we are sleeping, we are healing, recharging, generating new cells, and losing weight.

Sleep is almost more effective than fitness and diet combined.

You can fast for days and you will be ok with no food, you can go years without fitness, you will be ok not lifting a finger, but you can't function without sleep.

We must sleep to recharge, otherwise we quite literally will turn into a mad person.

Did you know 98% of fat burning happens while you are asleep? Something to think about right? Read that again, let it sink in. I'm sure I've got your full attention now! According to Ben Azadi (founder of Keto Kamp) research during delta sleep, where we activate our top 5 fat burning hormones. Which are, T3, Human Growth Hormone, IGF-1, Glucagon, and Testosterone. Delta sleep is further defined in Segen's Medical Dictionary as the deepest form of sleep, which is greatest in children and declines with age; it is thought that tissue repair and regeneration occur most efficiently during delta sleep.

This is why sacrificing sleep to get up early and exercise is a failing formula, so, just like children instinctively do, we need to trust our bodies and wake up when we wake up. Your body knows best. It may take some schedule adjusting and there will be a transitioning period, but the benefits are undeniably worth it.

We shouldn't exercise to lose weight, we should exercise to be fit and strong, you have a blank canvas to build and shape your body the way you want. It's up to you. **Weight loss is a side effect of being healthy, not a goal.**

Once you get healthy, weight will come off, Keto is not a diet, it is a lifestyle.

I personally don't eat anything that comes in a box, or is from a factory. I eat what is found in nature, I don't count calories, or worry about weight gain, because I know whatever I put in my body is good for me. It's also a mental attitude, if you believe it's good for you then it's good for you, if you are cheating and knowing that what you are eating is bad for you and think no one will know if you cheat, the most important part is that you know, your heart knows, therefore it's bad for you, you can't hide from your own self. It's time to get real.

No one cares for what you eat, you owe no explanations to anyone else but you do owe it to yourself to treat your entire being with love, confidence and honesty.

Here Are Some Tips For Good Sleep

Now that you are transitioning into a keto lifestyle and you are a fat burner, your body is running on fat for energy. Cutting down carb intake lowered your insulin production, which your brain was used to. Your brain will not adjust overnight. It's a process. You may lose sleep, you may have a busy mind, and not only will it be hard to fall asleep, you will find it equally difficult to stay asleep. This was especially the case with me. I would wake up in the middle of the night and feel like going for a run. So, I would watch the time instead, eagerly waiting until it was an appropriate hour to get up and have my coffee.

When I was new to keto, I probably watched all of the Keto Kamp YouTube videos, (thank you again Ben Azadi) he really did his homework! I used every tip he gave and followed all his recommendations. As you all know, I'm not reinventing the wheel here, this information is already out there, I am only sharing what worked for me.

Here are some of Ben's sleep tips.

Turn Your Bedroom Into A Sleep Cave

This one is my favorite, and it worked magic for me. When I started fasting, I had so much extra time because I wasn't cooking or washing dishes, or food shopping all the time. And it gave me extra time and money. So I started to clean out everything, anything I hadn't used for more than two years was either trashed or donated.

After I cleaned my bedroom along with the few other rooms that make up my home, my small apartment no longer seemed so small. Things had been congested, not only in my peace of mind but in my physical surroundings as well. You know what I mean, after removing all of the disorderly items merely taking up space, my room started breathing again, and I could feel the energy. It definitely shifted, all the old things that had been holding expired energy were gone, and what was left was like taking a deeper breath every time I walked in.

This opened up a tangible and beautiful emptiness patiently waiting to be filled with new energy. I feel so much peace and am deeply connected to the regenerated heartbeat of my home.

My next cleansing effort was to get rid of all electronics from my room. I got light blocking curtains. No WIFI, no phone, no lights, no laptop. I won't enter my room for at least 30 min before bed. And when I do go in for the night, I usually light my little candle and my room is prepared for me to sleep. I definitely journal before bed, whatever is on my mind will go in my notebook. It's more like a mental prep for me. You don't have to follow this routine if it doesn't resonate with you.

Another thing I learned is to keep my room in cool temperature, like 62 to 68F. This helps you to burn more fat, believe it or not, and you will stay asleep better.

Avoid Blue Light

This one is huge, because blue lights mess with your cortisol and melatonin. Blue light lowers your melatonin production, which you need to sleep. An hour before bed you can use blue light blocking glasses. **I use Ra Optics brand***

Supplements For Good Sleep

* Magnesium (400mg)
* Potassium (400 mg)
* MCT Oil (1 tablespoon)
* This is the best hack ever. This will cut all your nighttime cravings.

Raw Organic Honey

Oh, I know this is not keto. But this is not for someone who is fully transitioned; this is for someone still at the 21-28 day mark where they are still transitioning into keto. Our brain needs to adjust, and it can get hard at first, our brain is so used to using sugar (insulin) and now as the insulin is cut down it goes into shock, and it can't rest, so when this happens, you can take a teaspoon of raw honey, but did you read it well, I said a teaspoon. And this is not everyday, this is only when you are just transitioning. Don't make it a habit, because otherwise you won't be burning fat while asleep.

This Is A No! No!

Do not snack before bed. This is the worst thing you can do. It will mess up all the good work you have done all day, you need at least a 3-4 hour gap between your last meal and sleep, when you snack before bed, your body will be busy digesting the food you just ate, and not have time to burn fat or heal, or produce any anti-aging and healing hormones. Don't sabotage your progress; trust me it'll all get better, and these little discomforts will all pass.

Meditation

This is my favorite time of the day, time alone ☺. There are many ways to meditate; not necessarily sitting crossed legged and burning sage and candles while you "Om" your way into ascension. Time alone, time alone, time alone, I can't emphasize it enough, listening to a song, closing your eyes, listening to your heart's inner voice, and imagination. Go to a place in your mind where you can see everything clearly, and stay there, you will feel a smile coming to your face.

As I mentioned previously, I love **Dr. Joe Dispenza**, he has many meditation tools, and his book, Breaking the Habit of Being Yourself is literally my bible. I have it on my bed end table, I have it on Audio, and I listen and listen. Please get this book, it will teach you so much.

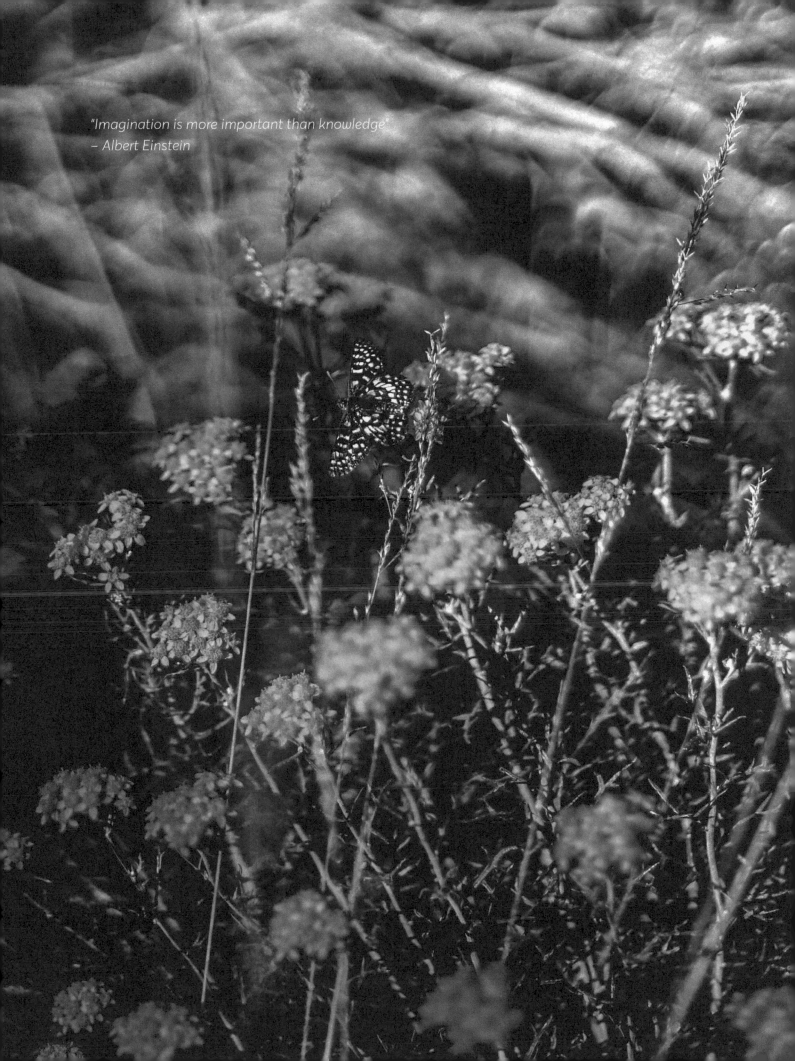

"Imagination is more important than knowledge"
– Albert Einstein

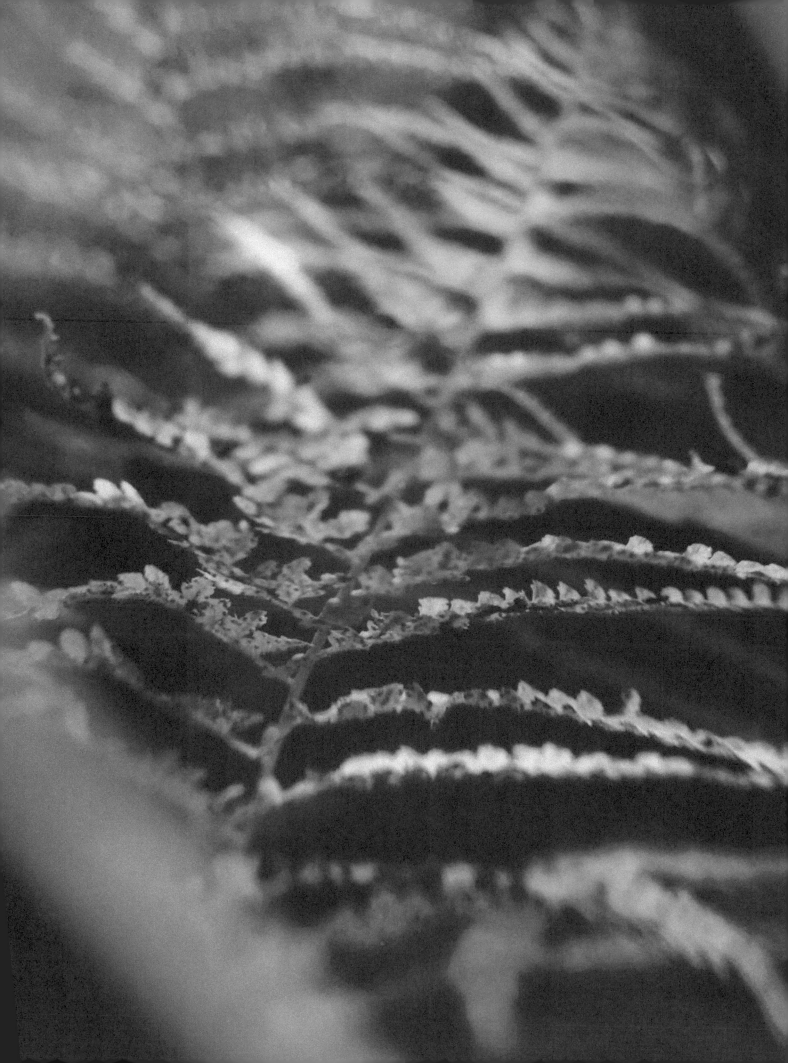

Imagination Creates The Feelings,
Feelings Creates The Vibrations,
Vibrations Creates The Reality

Julyet B.

CHAPTER 5

FASTING

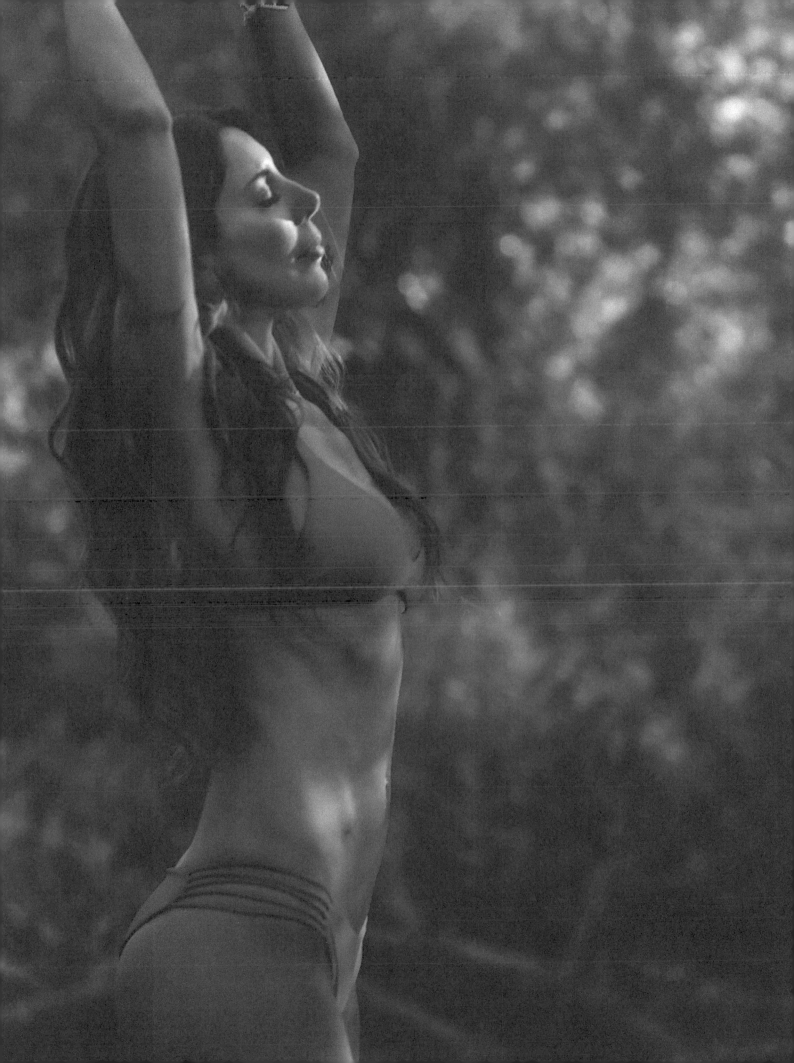

FASTING

Eeek, this is my favorite subject! As I start this chapter, I am 2.5 days into my fast. I'm going for 3 days.

Fasting is the best thing you can give to your body for detox and healing. Our body is a very smart machine. If given the opportunity, it will do magic for you. Think like this, you are forced to stay home for 3 days; you have no phone, no Internet and no one visiting you. You are all alone and after taking long naps, pacing around the house, you start getting bored, you will sit on your couch and start looking around, you will start seeing all the things that need your attention. You will start cleaning deep into the drawers you didn't pay attention to before. You ignored them for so long. You will start fixing things; you will be so busy taking care of your house that at the end of 3 days you will be surprised how much you've gotten done.

Fasting the body is the same. You usually feed your body every 2-3 hours, so this means it never gets the break it needs. Do you know how much energy it takes to digest food? A LOT ... *Your body will get a break now and it doesn't have to consistently digest the food you keep feeding it. Now it has time to sit back and look around.

Every 2-3 hours, your brain will automatically start sending signals to eat. Because you are programmed this way, now your body is expecting to be fed. These are hard habits but we create them, therefore we can create new ones.

Now you decided you wouldn't give food to your body every 2-3 hours, you want to fast for 16-18 hours, (by skipping a breakfast only) and this is your first try.

How Excited Are You To Start?

Let's get started!

So what happens to your body when only doing an 18 hour fast? Are you ready to be mind blown?

When you don't eat around the 16-18 hour mark, your glycogen stored in your liver becomes depleted. The body then switches from using sugar as a source of energy to using your body's fat. You can also get to this stage by exercising a lot.

This metabolic state is called KETOSIS and this brings about change in the body fast.

It is not a common practice to reach this state here in Northern America because we grew up hearing our moms telling us not to go to school on an empty stomach because our brains won't work. I remember this very well, like yesterday. Well … thanks mom!!!!

We have a lot of stored energy in our bodies as fat, old fat, stored in there for emergencies. This is from way back in the days when we were unable to hunt. Our bodies were built to sustain us for days without eating because our brain is a survival machine and it directs energy to be stored for the times it is impossible to find available sources of energy, aka food. Unfortunately, our brain (programming) is from a gazillion years ago (yes, that's the scientific consensus!) It still doesn't understand that we have Whole Foods next door, or any app will deliver food to our door in 20 min.

We also hold lots and lots of cells in those stored fats junk cells, they have no business staying around, they are disease causing, super aging, mind fogging little monsters.

So in ketosis our body uses the stored fat for energy, this is why you see a rapid change in such a short time. It is important to acknowledge that ketosis is the default human metabolic state; because it was the only way humans were able to survive during primal times.

Ketogenic eating can also protect against assorted inflammatory conditions that lead to dysfunction and disease like heart disease, cancer, and cognitive decline. When you are in the fasting stage your body goes into autophagy.

Autophagy is the body's way of cleaning out damaged cells, in order to regenerate newer, healthier cells.

"Auto" means self and "phagy" means eat. So the literal meaning of autophagy is "self-eating."

It's also referred to as "self-devouring." While that may sound like something you never want to happen to your body, it's actually beneficial to your overall health.

This is because autophagy is an evolutionary self-preservation mechanism through which the body can remove the dysfunctional cells and recycle parts of them toward cellular repair and cleaning.

The purpose of autophagy is to remove debris and self-regulate back to optimal smooth functioning.

It is recycling that's that and cleaning at the same time, just like hitting a reset button to your body. Plus, it promotes survival and adaptation as a response to various stressors and toxins accumulated in our cells.

At the cellular level, the benefits of autophagy include:

- Removing toxic proteins from the cells that are attributed to neurodegenerative diseases, such as Parkinson and Alzheimer's
- Recycling residual proteins
- Providing energy and building blocks for cells that could still benefit from repair
- On a larger scale, it prompts regeneration into the production of healthy cells

Autophagy is receiving a lot of attention for the role it may play in preventing or treating cancer.

The most, and I do mean the most important is that you get beautiful skin, and no wrinkles. Basically it's as though you stop aging - like it slows down massive amounts. Can you believe I'm over 40? Now that's real talk.

And the best part is you can start slowly and build yourself up to a full day of fasting, then 2 days, then 3, and it keeps getting better. Besides the fat loss, now you have added anti-aging, and disease prevention. Basically, now you can live longer, look younger even as you age (it's literally just a number), have more energy, because you keep cleaning the junk out of your system due to the lack of clogging you've induced with ketosis.

Taking this initial step of getting the junk out of your body is a huge deal. I am so excited for you and you will feel and look amazing in such a short time.

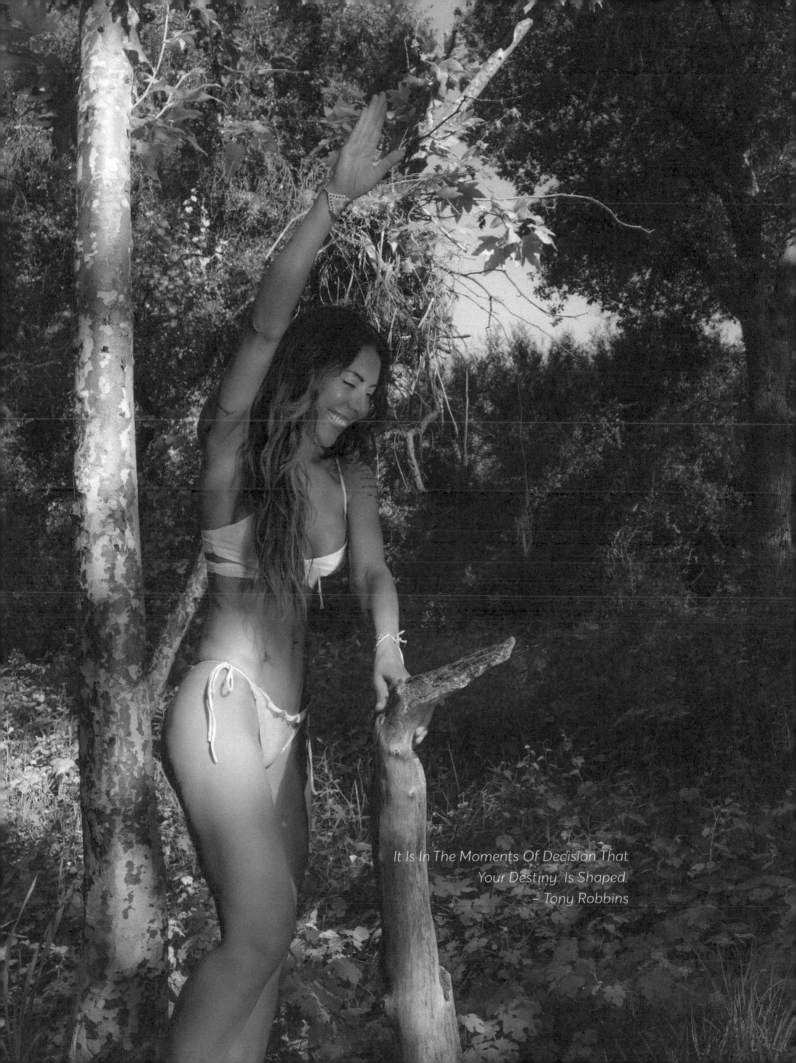

It Is In The Moments Of Decision That
Your Destiny Is Shaped.
– Tony Robbins

I promise you, you will never look back. Remember, your diet is as good as your last meal.

You will feel more energy, more alert, less hungry, less stress, and experience virtually no up's & down's.

You are finally going to use your body to its full potential by introducing fasting, and keto diet - now watch, just watch your body thrive.
We're not just talking about mere weight loss but also longevity, and did I mention no wrinkles?

Before we get started, I want you to ask yourself. What is your WHY? Why are you doing this? While the benefits are without a doubt worth it, this is still going to be a challenge in the beginning while we work to adjust your body composition. When you feel like giving up, I want you to go to your journal and read your WHY. Your WHY will be your best friend, it will help you keep your eye on the prize, and make sure you are brutally honest with your WHY.

This is only for you, not for anyone else. It's your time now, and only yours.
Giving up sugar dependency is not going to be easy, you will fail, and it's ok, you are supposed to fail, I know this because I failed four times before I actually fasted for even just one day.

Imagine you never worked out in your life and you are watching a cross fit video on YouTube and you said, ok I'm going to do this, you are all pumped up, you put your leggings on, and now you are ready rock.

Within 5 minutes max, if you even get that far, your heart will be pounding harder than your body can take, you will be out of breath and the worst part is you will be feeling completely defeated. But give yourself some credit and time. You will get there eventually.

There is no way you can master cross fit in a day and fasting is the same. I don't care how much willpower you have. You will fail. Your brain is in charge and you are not yet there in terms of controlling the power of your brain. You have to understand it first. You have to give your body a chance to adapt to a new way, and you may still fail, but it won't be as bad as your first fail.

The beauty is that you know where you are going and it's ok to tumble on the way, because your WHY is bigger than your little tumbles. Remember everything starts with the decision, and the determination for your well-being.

First, we will start by cleaning out your kitchen. I believe the kitchen is the heart of the home, I want you to get a garbage bag, go to your pantry and toss out everything in boxes, every wheat product, if it's not made in nature, you don't want to put it in your body. We don't get factory made foods. That's right. Get used to it. You're going to love me for it soon.

You especially want to be sure to rid your pantry of all the oils you've been using for cooking, Canola oil, Sunflower oil, Corn oil, vegetable oil, margarines, toss, toss, toss…

They are so inflammatory and so bad for you. Most diseases manifest because our physical bodies are inflamed on a cellular level, and these oils that I'm telling you to throw away, they contain Omega 6 which raises blood pressure and can potentially lead to blood clots resulting in heart attack and stroke. On a less severe level, omega 6 also causes your body to retain water and bloat and increases the likelihood of sleepless nights or insomnia.

Now you may wonder, what is there to eat once we toss out everything we used to eat. Not to worry, we're getting there and I will cover all of that for you.

Here is your new shopping list:

Broth

Bone broth, (recipe on chapter 6)

Full-Fat Dairy & Butter

- Goat Cheese
- Parmesan
- Cream
- Eggs
- Ghee
- Greek Yogurt
- Grass Fed Butter

Oils

- Avocado Oil
- Coconut Oil
- Mct Oil
- Olive Oil
- Macadamia Oil
- Sesame Oil

Flour & Baking Ingredients

- Almond Flour
- Coconut Flour
- Almond Meal
- Psyllium Husks
- Pepper
- Salt
- Spices
- Xanthan Gum

Nuts & Seeds

- Almond
- Brazil Nuts
- Chia Seeds
- Flaxseed
- Hazelnuts
- Hemp Hearts
- Macadamia Nuts
- Pecans
- Pine Nuts
- Pumpkin Seeds
- Sunflower Seeds
- Walnuts

Beverages

- Coffee
- Tea
- Water

Protein

- Bacon
- Chicken
- Fish
- Lamb
- Turkey
- Pork
- Prosciutto
- Seafood
- Shellfish
- 100% Grass-Fed, Grass-Finished Beef/Meats

Non-Starchy Veggies & Fruits

- Asparagus
- Avocados
- Bell peppers
- Blueberries
- Raspberries
- Broccoli
- Brussels sprouts
- Cabbage
- Carrots
- Celery
- Cucumber
- Garlic
- Green beans
- Kale
- Lettuce
- Spinach
- Olives
- Onion
- Tomato
- Zucchini

Treats & Sweeteners

- Dark Chocolate
- Cocoa Powder
- Erythritol
- Monk Fruit
- Stevia
- Xylitol

Now you have your new shopping list. This new kitchen is going to help you stay on track when you feel like cheating.

When you want to build a new habit your new behavior requires conscious planning, decision-making and self-control. The right products in your kitchen will help you succeed.

PREPARATION FOR FASTING

Journaling

Now before you start your fast, I want you to begin journaling. Devote 2-3 days of writing down and keeping track of what you're currently consuming. This way you will get a good idea of what your eating habits are before you change them entirely. Once we identify those, the rest will be so much easier to plan out. You will be surprised when you start recording your meal data at how unconscious we live on a day-to-day basis when it comes to putting food into our bodies. It's like we are on autopilot. Which you are, or you were up until just now.

You will be surprised at the amount of sugar and carbs you have been consuming. We won't immediately cut them out of your diet entirely but we will gradually lower your intake for a couple of days before your first fast.

For example, if you are having two pieces of toast for breakfast, begin by eating only one. Do the same for lunch, eating half portions of your carbs and sugars, getting your body used to the change, rather than drastically cutting them out completely. The carb intake will raise your insulin production which is sugar and your body uses that for energy but it's short lived, therefore you need to eat so often to keep the body going, so many ups and downs, It's like putting little pieces of wood in a fire all throughout the day, having to rekindle that fire constantly. With the keto diet, on the other hand, it's like you're placing one huge, slow burning log into a fire and then it burns all day, fueling your body and giving you energy so that you don't feel hunger or the mood swings that come with it. You will also start drinking more water. I prefer a gallon a day, (not to worry, you will get there).

We are not rushing you into fasting because we want long lasting results and we want to make sure it's sustainable with little to no discomfort. The changes will be permanent. This is not a diet book, KETO is a lifestyle. It's a metabolic process. Our goal is to move away from being an insulin burner to a fat burner body.

After you repeat lowering carb intake for breakfast, lunch and dinner, I would like you to stop eating after 6 pm, make sure you have at least 4-5 hours between your last meal and sleep. If you eat too close to sleep time, you won't be able to sleep, because your body will be so busy digesting and it needs energy for that so it will keep producing energy and your sleep will be ruined. Sleep, as I've already stressed in the "What is Keto" portion of your book, is the most important part of our health.

It's so important, I'll say it again, a lot happens while we are sleeping, the body regenerates and heals and most weight loss happens while we are asleep. You want to give your body the maximum opportunity and not interfere with it.

Now let's get back to fasting prep. After lowering your carb intake for a couple of days, you will feel lighter, you probably lost some water weight, because as you know carbs makes our bodies retain water, but now the water has nothing to stick to so it leaves the body, the reason we up the water intake is that we don't get dehydrated, when you start losing water you will also lose electrolytes, which will cause for you to feel hunger, get dizzy upon standing up fast, and feel tired. But this is a quick fix, electrolyte loss comes from low sodium, this is cellular dehydration, by replacing the sodium, you will get rid of this problem. I usually put a teaspoon of Himalayan salt into my water, and if I still feel dizzy. I put some salt under my tongue. You will find the recipe for the morning cocktail (see chapter 6). By replacing electrolytes, you will eliminate keto-flu. Which happens from loss of sodium and potassium. In the morning cocktail, we cover both. Please don't skip your morning cocktail. Taking it will set you up for success.

Now, you are ready to go for 18 hours with no food. I'm so proud of you for getting this far already; half of the battle is done. I get butterflies when my friends start this way and text me with great news. You can't see me now but while I'm writing this I have a massive grind on my face.

Our plan now is to try the 18/6 schedule. Which means, you stop eating by 6 pm, then resume eating the next day at noon.

Let's say you woke up at 6am(that's usually when I wake up) and you are going to skip breakfast (a little FYI, BREAK-FAST means what it says: a break from fasting, BREAK-FAST) you will delay it today until 12 noon.

First thing you do is to go to the bathroom, brush teeth, scrape tongue, pee, clean up, weigh yourself and write it down. Now we have a starting point.

Next, you prep your morning cocktail. (see chapter 6) you drink that, after you can have your bulletproof coffee *(see chapter 6)*.

Bulletproof coffee will feed your Mitochondria, which generates most of the energy needed to power the cell's biochemical reactions. These little powerhouse cells take the food you eat and the air you breathe and turn them into energy.

Bulletproof coffee has MCT oil and Grass-fed butter added in it, which gets you into ketosis in minutes and provides abundant fuel for your mitochondria. Ketones boost your metabolism, increase fat burning, curb your hunger, and sharpen your focus.

Now this will help you skip breakfast and keep going until 12 noon, but let's say you are feeling hungry, and it's 11 am, you don't know if you can hold on (side note: I know you can), let's say, it's unbearable and you feel you are about to fail. Here's another hack for you to keep going.

ARTISANA, this is my favorite brand of raw, organic, non-GMO coconut butter. It's magic. Yes, magic. Now, grab a spoonful. Yup, just like that. Now drink some water to wash it down.

Next, trick to help abate that hunger is to put a pinch of salt under your tongue and wait to feel what begins to happen. You just fed the brain what it needed; now it will leave you alone. This way now you can go until break-fast time, don't be surprised if you are not feeling hungry at break-fast time, then keep going. Don't eat just because it's "time to eat," eat when you are ready, once you've finished your ketosis, you used fat as energy, you know you lost fat. Now you feel like a winner, it's time to eat.

But, what do you eat, right? Well, lucky you, I have included amazing recipes for you in this book. They are super simple and keto friendly. You will enjoy preparing your food because you'll be doing it with love, you will smell and taste each ingredient deeply, since we started cleaning the body, it is now reaching its full potential.

Now, let's continue this 18/6 for another week, you will see at this point, weight is coming off rapidly, you can lose up to 2lbs a day.

What happens next as you continue this way, is that you become insulin sensitive. What does that mean for you?

Insulin sensitivity describes how sensitive the body is to the effects of insulin. When you are insulin sensitive, it will require smaller amounts of insulin to lower blood glucose levels than someone who has low sensitivity.

WHY IS INSULIN SENSITIVITY IMPORTANT?

Low insulin sensitivity can lead to a variety of health problems. The body will try to compensate for having a low sensitivity to insulin by producing more insulin. However, a high level of circulating insulin is associated with damage to blood vessels, high blood pressure, heart disease, heart failure and obesity, osteoporosis and even cancer.

Since your body doesn't get its energy from insulin anymore, when it receives insulin, it won't need as much as before, because you cut the life line. So, when you eat, you will feel full faster. Now, let's look into Leptin.

What is Leptin?

Leptin is your "stop eating" hormone, it tells your brain when you're full and controls your appetite and energy expenditure, which can decrease fat stores and help you with weight loss.

When leptin is working properly, when your cells are leptin sensitive, leptin helps you stay lean and healthy, but high levels of leptin from eating a poor diet, especially one high in sugar, can lead to leptin resistance.

When you're leptin resistant, you start a vicious cycle of putting on fat mass, which is why obesity researchers are looking at leptin resistance as one of the main roadblocks in weight management.

How Does Leptin Work?

When you eat food, fat cells send leptin to your hypothalamus, a part of your brain that controls appetite. When leptin reaches your brain, it shuts down hunger. The more leptin reaches your brain, the more full you feel.

Leptin also affects the reward center of your brain. It controls dopamine in the nucleus accumbens, the part of your brain that responds to pleasure.

That means the more leptin there is, the less rewarding food becomes. Leptin shuts down your motivation to keep eating, which is why dessert stops being so appealing after you have already had a helping or two.

Finally, leptin boosts energy expenditure by increasing the rate at which you burn fat. BINGO!

How does keto diet play a role in all this?

The ketogenic diet decreases hunger through several mechanisms.

A keto diet:

- Decreases circulating levels of ghrelin, the hormone that makes you hungry
- Boosts a hormone called cholecystokinin, or CCK, which binds to the hypothalamus to reduce hunger
- Reduces levels of neuropeptide, a brain factor that stimulates appetite Keto aligns your hormones so that you feel satisfied with less food.

I don't want to bore you with all these scientific explanations but as I was first starting out, I was obsessed with knowing what was happening inside my body. I wanted to know why I had finally lost the hunger, I have tried every diet on the books and up until now nothing worked so fast, or lasted. That's why I would like for you to know the reasons behind your awesomeness, it is not an accident; it works because we are made for it.

At this stage you should be into week one or two and feeling great, lost some weight, so much energy and now you are ready to take it to the next level.

Yes, you heard me, next level. I'm talking about going without food for 24 hours. I am sure, this will be a piece of cake for you now, 24 hours can be done once you master 18 hours, and now you have the tools, also you have changed your hormones and you are in control of everything. A long period of fasting has amazing benefits to our body.

Once I had done 10 days, after many failures, (because I didn't have this book to help me get ready) the first 2 days were my hardest, but after that I'm being honest when I tell you, it was so easy.

Let me tell you what happens to your body when fasting for longer periods of time.

Day 1

After about 8 hours of fasting, the liver will use the last of its glucose reserves. Fasting mode then becomes starvation mode. At this point, your metabolism slows down, and you begin burning fat for energy.

Day 2-7

You feel less hungry and more energetic and this will last until day 7. A lot of changes begin to happen at this stage, and you may start to notice changes in your physical appearance, as well as how you feel.

Day 8-15

Stage three typically falls between day 8 and 15. This stage includes dramatic improvements in mood and mental clarity and is the stage I look forward to the most. It almost feels like you are high on life. So epic!
I usually do periodic prolonged fasting, only when I feel like it. Yes, I actually crave fasting now, it became my super power, funny enough, I feel I can fix anything with my body if I give it the chance to. My normal week is 5 days 18/6, 1 day 24 hour fast, 1 day I eat 3 meals, I try, I don't really get hungry anymore and my portions are way smaller.

When I feel like it, about every other week, I will go 3 days.

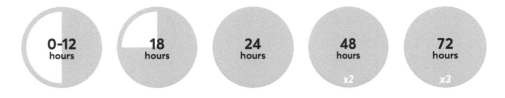

0-12 Hours ◐

Right about the 12-hour mark you get a spiking Growth Hormone (GH), which is the anti-aging hormone as well as the main fat burning hormone. Some people get this hormone injected. I like no risk and mine homemade, so I can produce it naturally and it's free. Did I mention no wrinkles ☺ The good part is it starts about the 12th hour and keeps increasing as you go on.

18ᵗʰ Hour

Now you entered the autophagy stage which I already explained in earlier pages, this is when the cleaning starts, getting rid of junk cells and renewing them.

24ᵗʰ Hour

Now you are running on ketones alone, which is the superior fuel for your body. Around the 24th hour mark your inflammation is greatly reduced, and if you add vitamin D this will increase the reduction even faster. At this stage you are also getting more gut healing because now your gut doesn't have to work so frequently. Also worth mentioning is that at this point you are producing more stem cells.

48ᵗʰ Hour

At this stage you are a stem cell producing machine, massive healing taking place and it's super anti-aging, while I'm writing this I kind of want to go another 3 days again, which I have just done.

I'm telling you, once you start, there is no going back, my body became my own science project, I appreciate it so much, I have so much gratitude and love towards my body.

72ⁿᵈ Hour

If you push it and go 72 hours. Not only are you healing by producing so many stem cells, you are also making your immune system stronger. To be honest I never get sick.

I'm seriously so proud of you for even buying this book. That means you are really looking for a change. Ketogenic lifestyle changed my life, and I'm so passionate about sharing it with everyone.

By going ketogenic your insulin production will get low, and your blood sugar will go down, you may feel light headed, hunger, cravings, and sometimes even headaches, but don't give up, these are temporary, and remember to always go back to your WHY.

All you need to do is drink the morning cocktail (chapter 6), increase potassium, sodium, apple cider/lemon will help with these symptoms so your journey is smoother.

And keep referring back to this book. It's your guide to make it through to the other side. YOU GOT THIS!

REFEEDING AFTER A PROLONGED FAST

This is one of the most important parts of your fast. How you break your fast is as important as how you prep for a fast.
Most people don't realize this until after it's too late, meaning, they gorge on food after fasting, and they get sick.

If you fasted for 3 days, you literally shut down the entire digestive system. You have to be careful not to shock your body by placing so much stress on your digestion, it by eating so much food. You also want to eat light food. Choosing things easy to digest. Our goal is not to put so much weight on our stomach. You have to start gradually.

It doesn't matter if you are a Ferrari or a Jeep, you can't turn the engine and shift it to fifth gear immediately, you have to gain momentum, it's exactly the same. You have to start from the first gear and start slow. If you follow the rules, you will have no problem going back to eating normal again.

Here is what I do after a prolonged fasting. I have never had any discomfort or problems.

When the time comes to break my 3 days fast, I will pick one kind of fruit that I will eat the first day, usually I like watermelon, at this stage I am not worried about staying in ketosis, I am getting out of ketosis.

I will have watermelon whenever I feel like eating, same thing all day. I won't mix any other food, just watermelon, day two I will eat steamed broccoli, add salads, and eggs. Eggs are the best kind of protein to introduce if you're breaking your fast, it's easy to digest. As usual I will drink at least a gallon of water, salt and lemon added. This helps with electrolytes.

Day 3, I will start eating as I usually eat. Once you go back to normal, you can start your 18/6 schedule again.

CHAPTER 6

FOOD IS MEDICINE

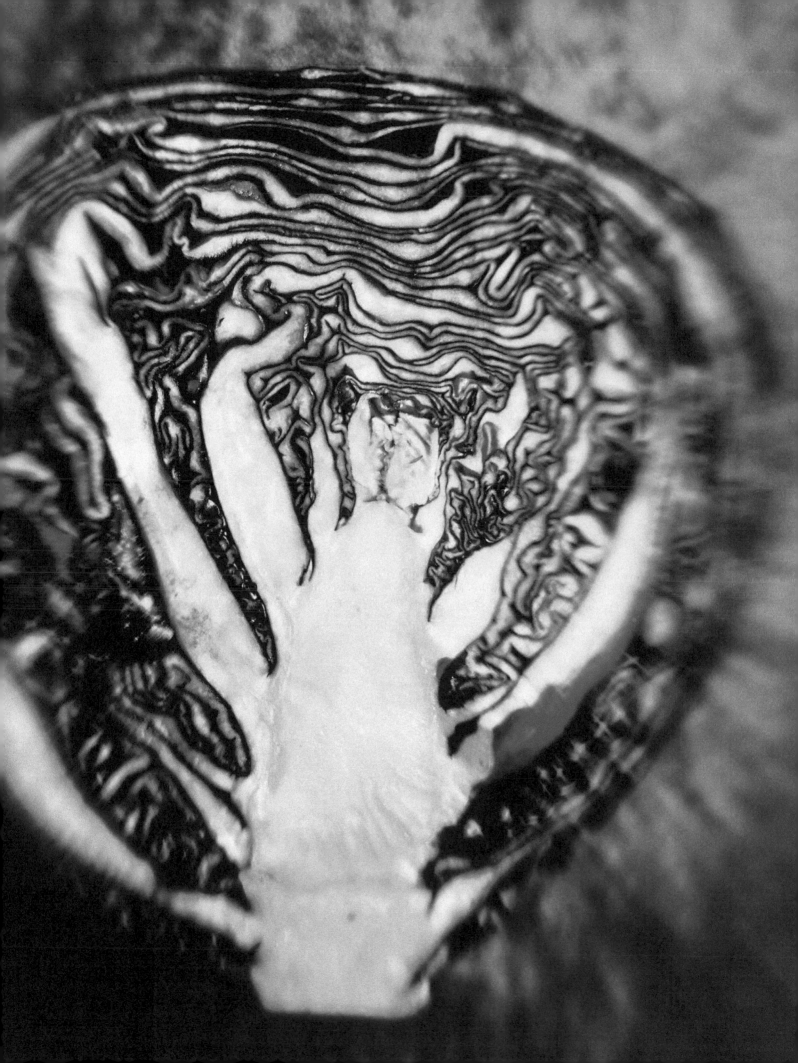

RECIPES INDEX

Menemen ... *119*

Spinach & Mushroom & Goat Cheese Omelette ... *120*

Julyet's Avocado Toast ... *123*

Burrata Salad ... *124*

Cabbage Taco ... *127*

Musakka ... *128*

Turkish Meatballs – Köfte ... *131*

Morning Cocktail ... *132*

Chicken Bone Broth ... *133*

Chopped Salad ... *134*

Grilled Lamb Chops ... *137*

My Butter Cup Of Joe ... *138*

Pom-Yo-Chai ... *141*

Salmon ... *143*

New York Steak ... *144*

Oh, how much I love cooking, I learned how to cook from my grandmother and my mother, I used to love hanging out in the kitchen with them, because that was the only time I get to have the longest time with them, Turkish women seems to spend a lot of time in the kitchen and I picked up a thing or two while hanging with my favorite women.

I am not a trained chef but I know many little tricks. Which I share with you here. I eyeball everything, I don't usually follow recipes, for that reason, I want to make all of these recipes for you so that they are easy to follow and implement.

My main ingredient and most important ingredient is LOVE. I love cooking and I love when people eat my food. It makes me so happy to see the face they make while they are eating. I know it sounds a bit selfish but it makes me happy to see them happy. It's healthy-selfish!.

Food brings families together, brings friends together. The best conversations always happen around a table with so much love.

My grandmother always said, if you know how to cook, you would never be hungry. I love knowing what I am eating; I am not a big fan of eating out. I want to know the details of the food. How it's been prepared. I know that makes me a bit of a snob, but hey, you are what you eat. Literally. And it is my every right to know what I am eating. What I am putting into my body and I take this very seriously.

I am sharing my favorite foods here with you. I prepare and eat all of them.

Everything you will find here is good for you and fits perfectly with your keto lifestyle. I also put some bread in there for Keto Flex days. Yes you can incorporate carbs, but healthy carbs on your keto flex days, which I usually do before my moon time. I use the 5 days window to get some carbs in, the ones I miss the most. Which is usually bread.

There are some adjustments I made. Instead of rice, I use quinoa. And for sugar I use monk fruit. You can also use stevia. I just don't like the taste so I use monk fruit. For flour replacement, I use cassava flour, or coconut flour, or almond flour. These are all safe to use.

I hope you enjoy making them and eating them and serving them as much as I do. All made with so much love and smile.

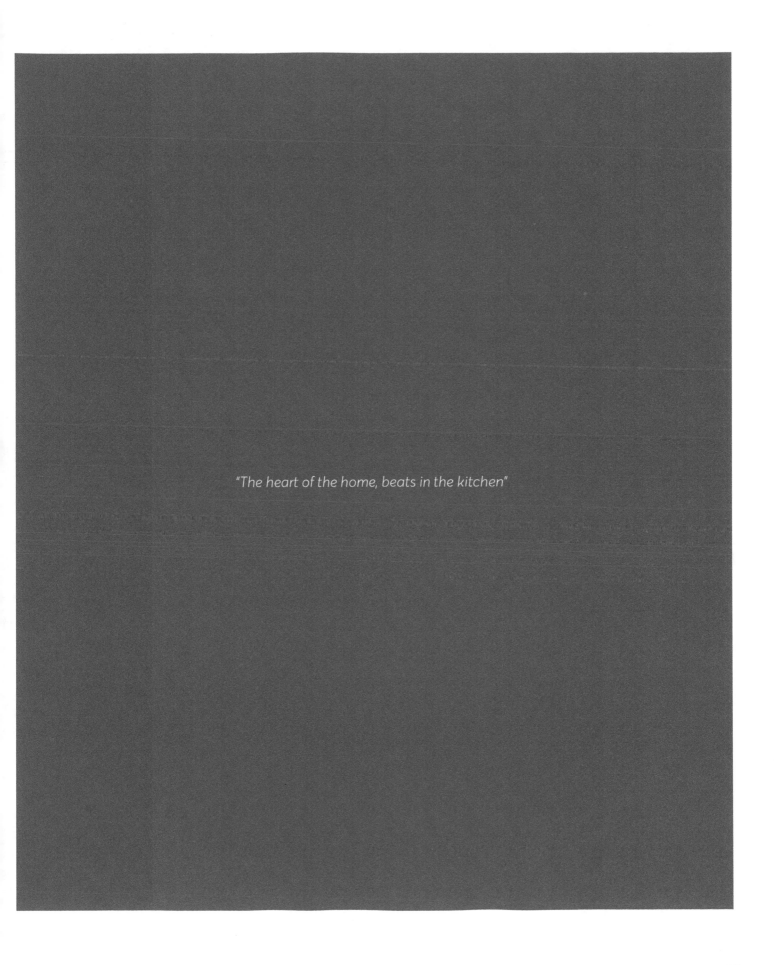

"The heart of the home, beats in the kitchen"

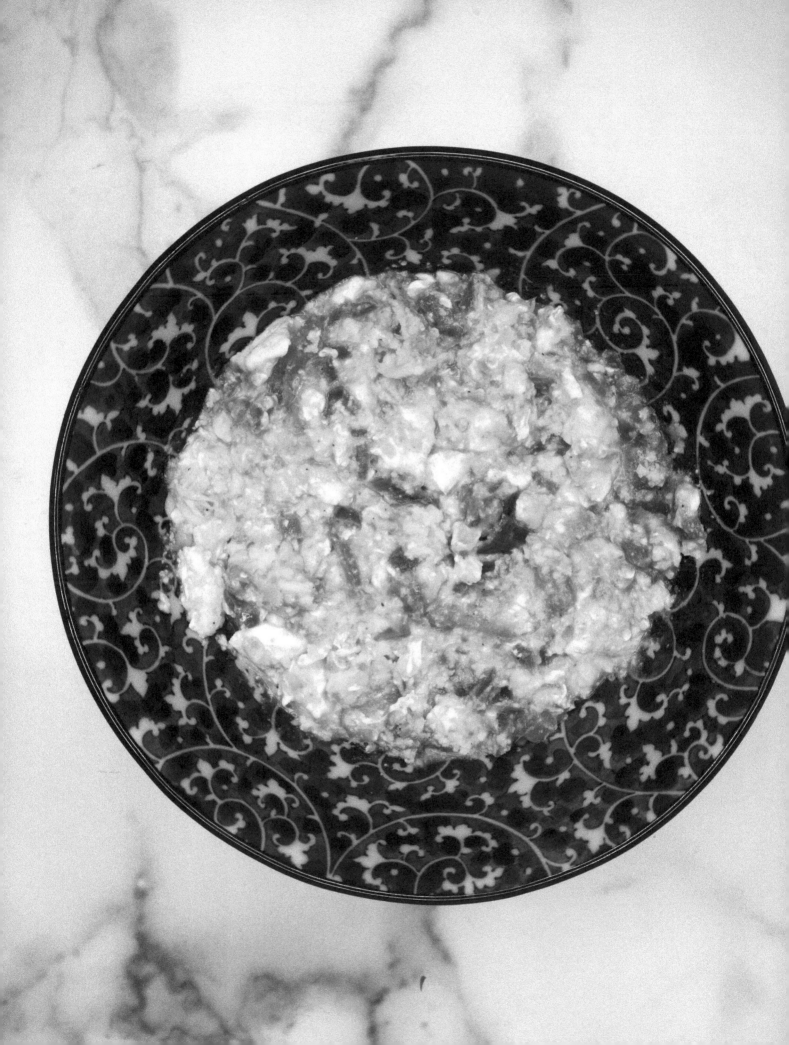

Menemen

You Need:

8 Eggs
1 Tablespoon Kerrygold Grass-Fed Butter
(salted)
2 Medium size Tomatoes
1 Medium size Anaheim Pepper
1 Teaspoon salt
1 Teaspoon black pepper
½ Cup crumbled feta cheese
½ Cup fresh Italian parsley

Side Options:

Fresh sliced tomatoes
½ avocado
Bacon

Prep :

Cut the Anaheim pepper in half and remove the seeds out. After you dice them into little pieces. Remove the tomatoes skin; I usually put the tomatoes in a hot water for a second to help remove the skin easier. Then dice them into small pieces as well. Chop the parsley. Break all the eggs in a bowl.

Heat your pan, melt the butter and add the Anaheim pepper first, let it cook a bit like 2 min, you will see that it will start to melt, add salt and black pepper, after add the diced tomatoes, let it cook until it gets thicker. I usually cook it for like 5 min until all the excess juice has evaporated. Add the eggs, feta and parsley now, with a fork, now start mixing it until it's cooked the way you like it. I like mine a bit softer, but you can cook it all the way.

And that's it.

I usually serve it with a side of avocado and some fresh sliced tomatoes and bacon. *Optional*

Enjoy.

Spinach & Mushroom & Goat Cheese Omelette

You Need:

3 Eggs
1 Cup of button mushrooms
1 Cup of organic spinach
1 Tablespoon of goat cheese
1 Tablespoon of Kerrygold grass-fed
butter (salted)
1 Teaspoon salt
1 Teaspoon black pepper

Side Options:

Bacon
Fresh sliced tomatoes
Fresh sliced cucumbers
Avocado

Prep:

For this you will need 2 pans. First let's start with slicing the mushrooms. Break your eggs into a bowl and mix them well, add the salt and pepper while mixing the eggs. In one pan, melt the butter and add the mushrooms. I like to toss them until they are golden, while your mushrooms are cooking on the other pan, start cooking your eggs. Now add the spinach with the mushrooms, toss them, then transfer all onto the eggs, add the goat cheese and flip half of the egg and cover the mushrooms and spinach and goat cheese and flip it.

That's it.

I serve it with the side of ½ avocado and fresh sliced cucumber and tomatoes. Yum.

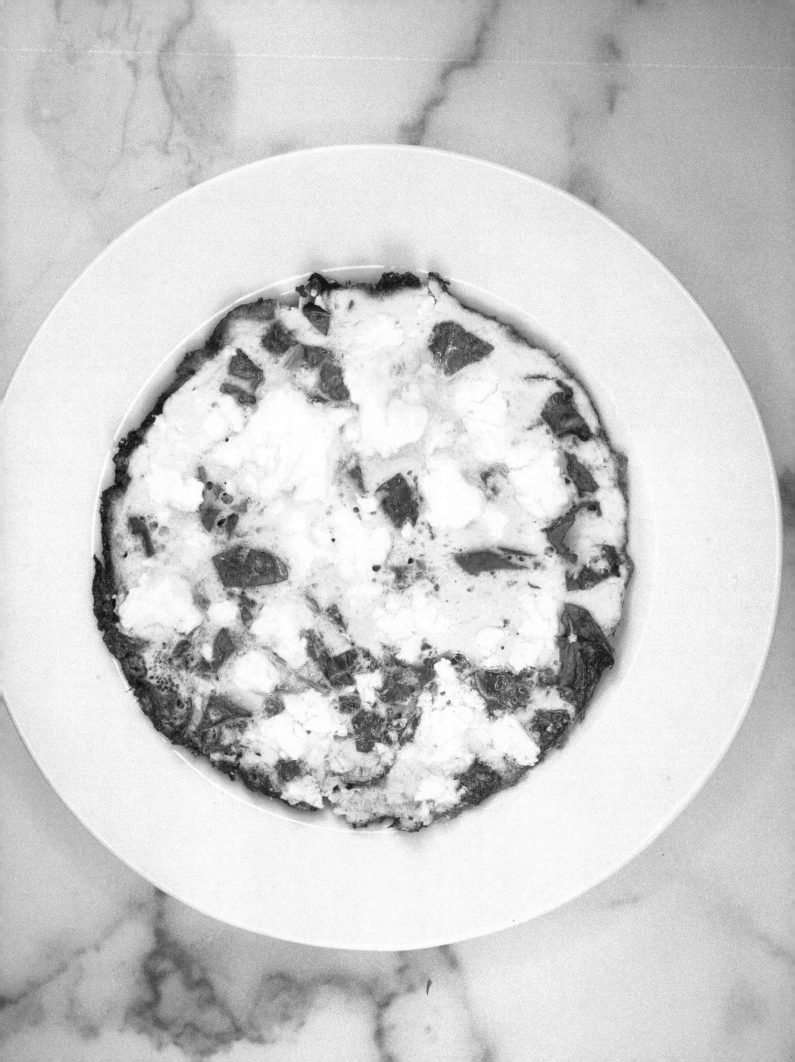

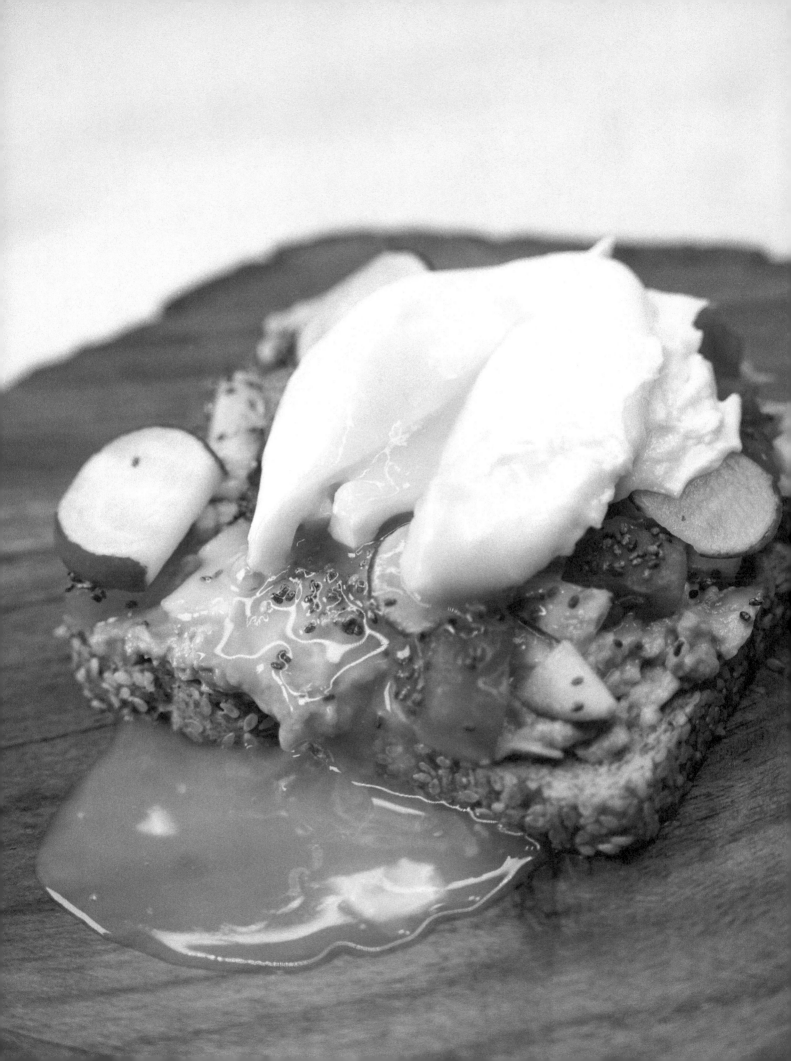

Julyet's Avocado Toast

You Need:

1 slice of sprouted sourdough bread is my choice but you can use gluten free option any of your favorite slice

Avocado
Egg
Cucumber
Tomato
Thin sliced radish
Lemon
Coarse sea salt
Black pepper
Olive oil
Chia seeds –optional–

I only eat bread on the day I don't fast and closer to my moon time, which I explained on fasting section.

Prep:

Toast your bread, while it's toasting, cut your avocado, smush it with a fork, add lemon and salt & pepper, and drizzle of olive oil.

Spread it over your toasted bread, thin sliced cucumber, radishes and tomato go on top, and sprinkle some chia seeds, this also gives that perfect crunch with each bite.

The final touch, place your poached egg on top.

Burrata Salad

You Need:

Burrata
Heirloom tomatoes
Basil
Olive oil
Vinegar
Black olives

Prep:

Pretty easy I say, just slice them all and place it on a plate, olive oil, vinegar, salt to taste. Enjoy...

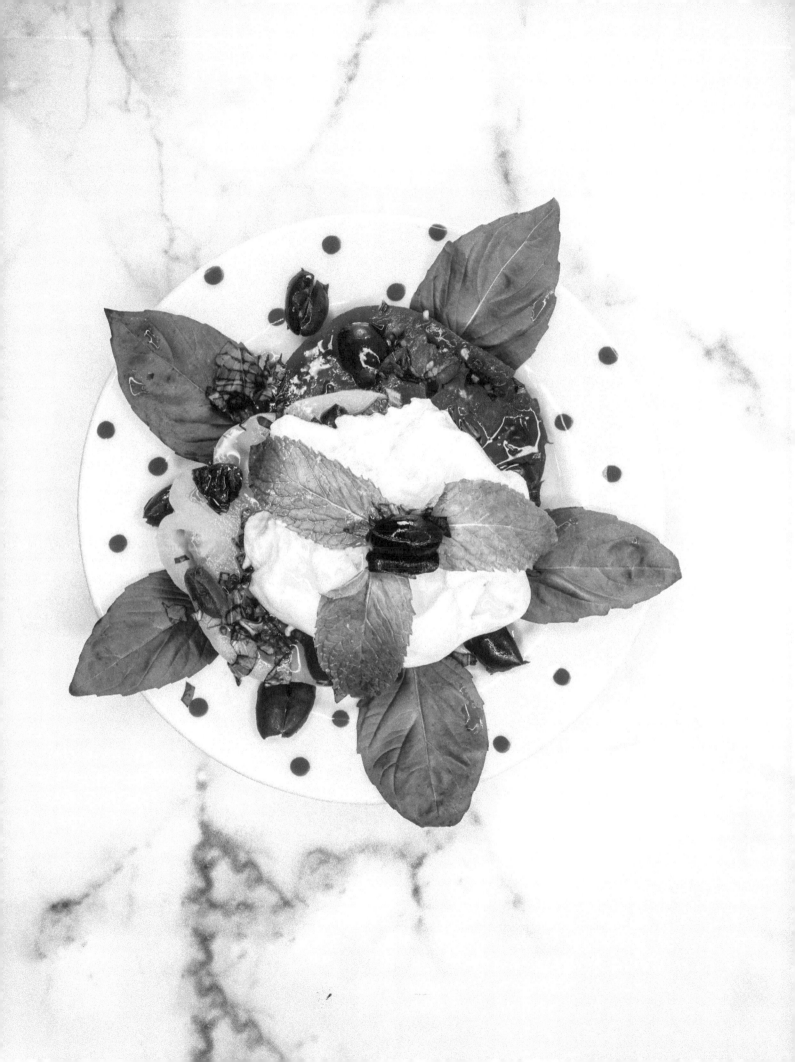

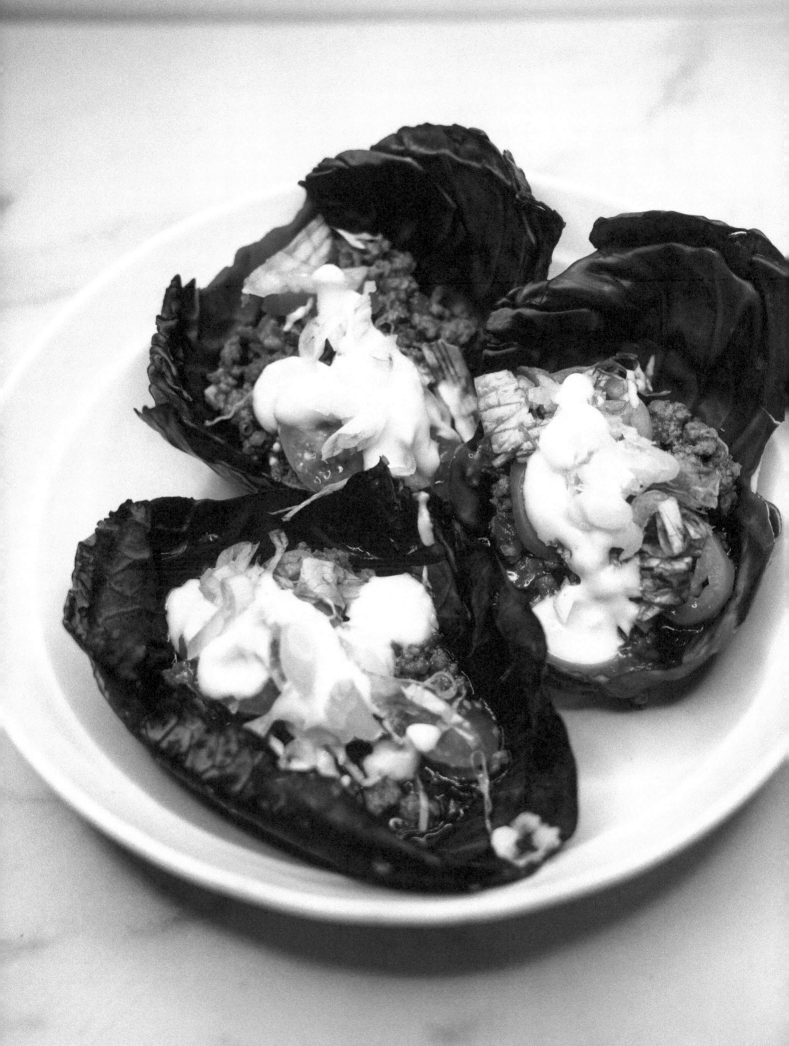

Cabbage Taco

You Need:

1 Red or White Cabbage
½ Ground beef (100% grass-fed, grass-finished)
2 Tomatoes
3 Garlic Cloves
1 Yellow Onion
1 Green Fresh Pepper

½ Cup Plain Yogurt
Salt & black pepper
½ cup Chicken Broth
Scallions
Avocado oil

Prep:

Dice tomatoes, scallion's onion and fresh green pepper and garlic into small pieces. Heat the avocado oil in a pan medium heat and add onion and green pepper, add salt and pepper, cook a bit until they are translucent and kind of melted after add the garlic, (garlic tends to burn fast if you add with the onion and pepper, so I always make sure I cook the onion and pepper first and after I add the garlic). Give it a good mix and add the ground beef, here you will need to mix them all together until the meat is semi cooked. Now add the diced fresh tomatoes, half a cup a chicken broth and let it simmer for like 10 min. you are pretty much done, I let it cool a bit, before I place it into a cabbage leaf so it doesn't melt the leaf.

After it cools down a bit, place a spoon full of meat into a leaf, on top I put thin slice scallions and spread a bit of yogurt on top. Hope you enjoy it as much as I do.

Musakka

You Need:

1 large eggplant
½ Ground beef (100% grass-fed,
grass-finished)
2 Tomatoes
3 Garlic Cloves

1 Yellow Onion
1 Green Fresh Pepper
Salt & black pepper
½ cup Chicken Broth
Avocado oil

Prep:

Little tip for the eggplant before we start anything

Cut the eggplant into decent size slices and place them into salted water, you can be generous with the salt, this will remove any bitterness from the eggplant and let the eggplant soak in the water while you prep the meat sauce. Once you remove the eggplants from the water you will see the water will be darker color. After dry your eggplants and set a side. Heat the avocado oil in high heat, fry the eggplants until both sides are a golden color, then place them on a paper towel for the excess oil to be removed.

For the meat sauce, heat the avocado oil in a pan on medium heat and add onion and green pepper, add salt and pepper, cook a bit until they are translucent and kind of melted after add the garlic, (garlic tends to burn fast if you add with the onion and pepper, so I always make sure I cook the onion and pepper first and after I add the garlic). Give it a good mix and add the ground beef, here you will need to mix them all together until the meat is semi cooked. Now add the diced fresh tomatoes, half a cup a chicken broth and let it simmer for like 10 min. you are pretty much done.

Now place all the eggplants on a cooking sheet, put a decent amount of meat on top. After that is done put it in the oven for 10 min. This way the juices from the meat sauce get into the eggplant. It's ready to serve. Enjoy!

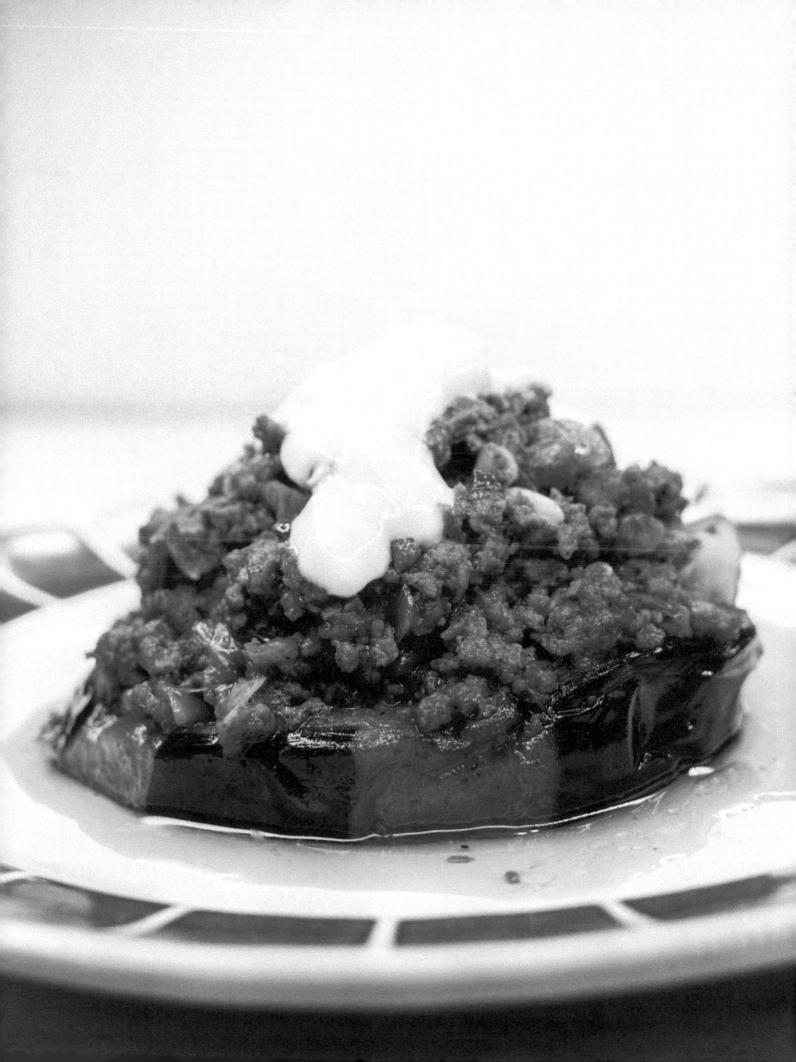

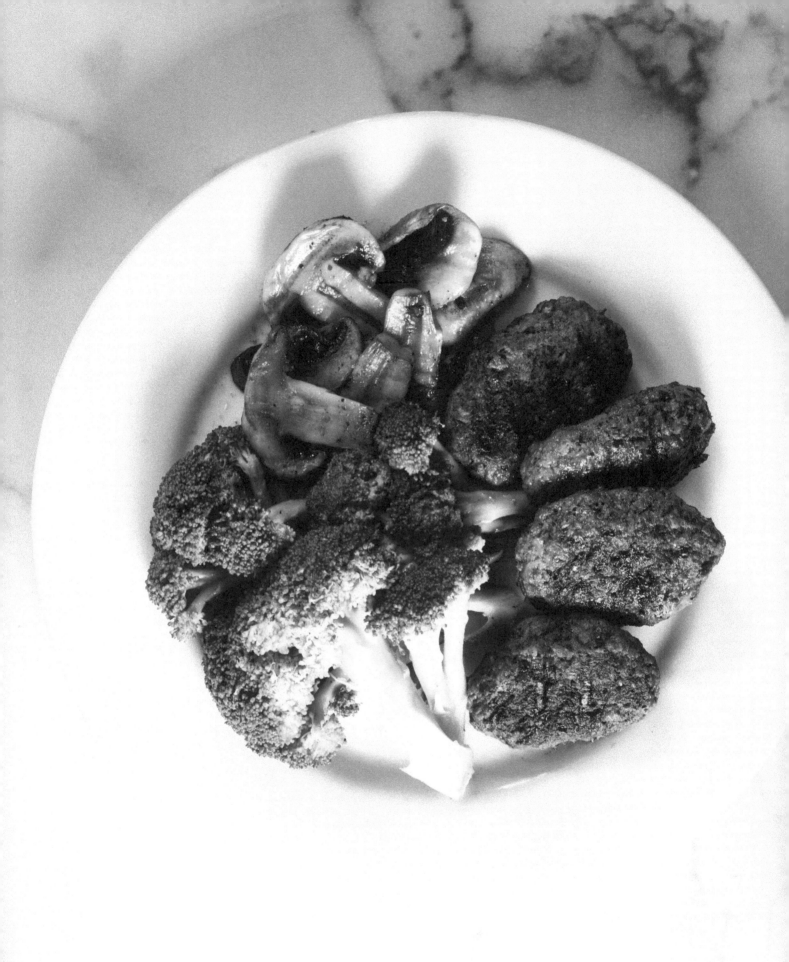

Turkish Meatballs – Köfte

You Need:

1 pound of ground beef - I prefer 80/20 fat ratio
1 yellow onion
Salt & pepper

1 Teaspoon of cumin
½ cup of fresh parsley
Avocado oil

Prep:

I usually grind the onion but if you want to avoid the tears, you can use a food processor. Cut the onion into chunks and put it into the food processor, add the fresh parsley as well. Add salt and pepper and cumin. Mix it all until it becomes like a paste.

Place the meat into a mixing bowl, add the paste, mix it and shape them into patties. Heat the avocado oil and fry them or you can grill them, however you would like to cook. In the traditional recipe, we add breadcrumbs to bind the meat together, I don't use any, but if you like, you can always use almond flour as a binder. Either works well.

You can serve the meatballs with any side dishes you desire.

Morning Cocktail

You Need:

Liter Water
Lemon Juice Squeezed
Teaspoon Himalayan Salt
Teaspoon Cream of Tartar

Prep:

Mix it all together; drink it first thing in the morning, when you wake up to eliminate dehydration.

Especially if you are fasting this will help you a lot. We tend to lose electrolytes while we are fasting, lack of carb intake makes us lose more water during fasting; carbs makes us hold more water in the body. That is why most people lose up to 5lbs of water weight the first week of their fast. This cocktail will replace your sodium and potassium, which means, you won't feel dizzy upon standing up, or feel hunger during your fast. Regardless, I drink this every morning. It is very good for your body and overall health.

Disclaimer: Before you start any kind of diet changes always check with your doctor to make sure it's ok for you.

Chicken Bone Broth

You Need:

4 Cups of chicken bones from 3 pounds of chicken

2 to 3 cups vegetable like one large onion with the skin roughly cut.

2 Celery stalks

2 Carrots roughly chopped.

2 Garlic cloves crushed

1 Tablespoon minced fresh ginger

10 Whole black peppercorns

1 Dried bay leaf

Fresh herbs such as thyme or rosemary spring (optional)

Prep:

Place all ingredients in a slow cooker with enough water to completely cover. Set heat low; cook it at least 8 hours. You can also cook it for 24 hours or more. **P.S.** This recipe I learned from Mark Sisson, it's one of my favorite bone broth.

Chopped Salad

You Need:

Tomato
Cucumber
Red onion
Parsley
Black olives
Olive oil
Lemon

Prep:

Super easy to prep and so delicious. Chop them all into little squares and mix with olive oil and lemon juice. That's it. Enjoy!

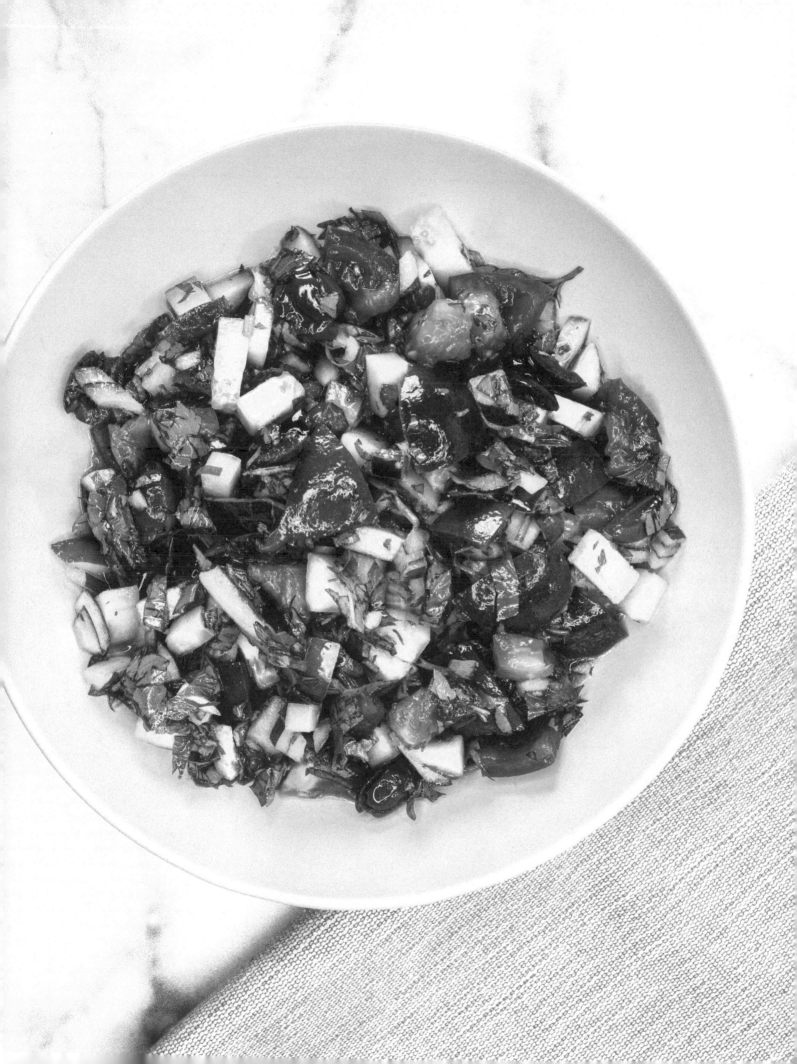

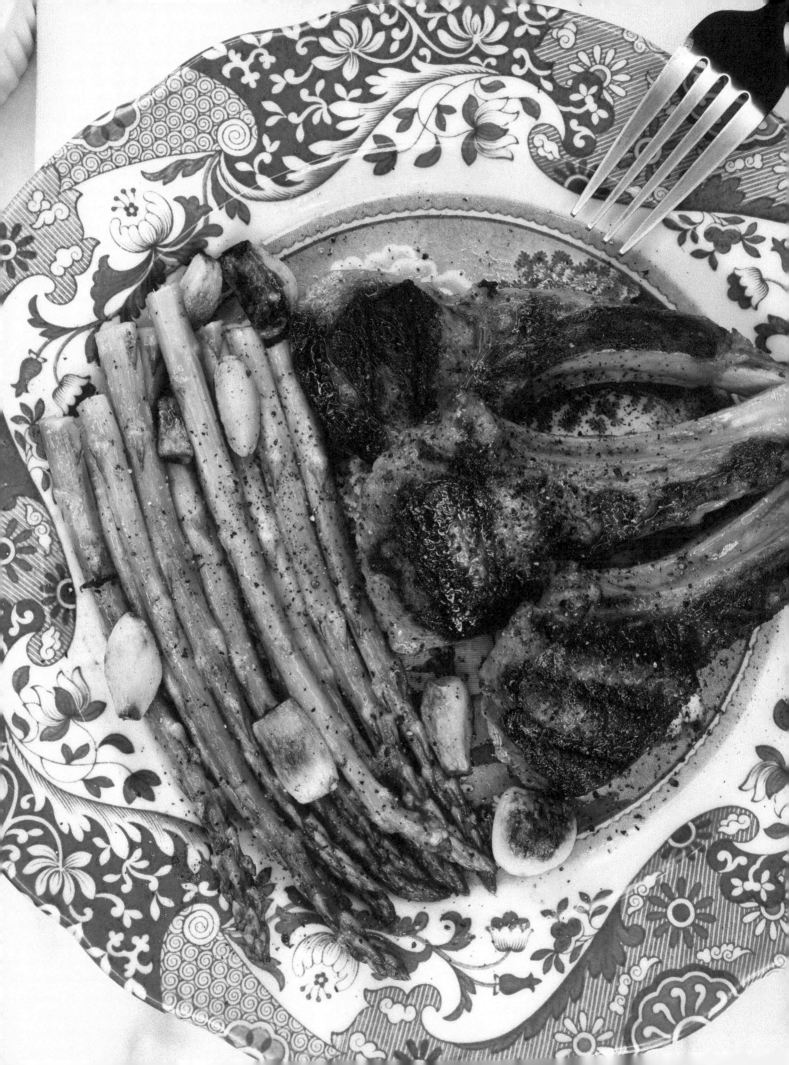

Grilled Lamb Chops

You Need:

8 Lamb chops
Juice of 1 lemon
¼ Olive oil
2 tablespoon dried oregano
4 cloves Garlic minced
1 tablespoon of salt
1 tablespoon avocado oil for cooking

Prep:

Using paper towels pat dry the chops. Mix all the ingredients together in a small bowl. Pour the marinade all over the lamb rubbing into the meat. Marinate it for 30 min., or you can marinate it overnight in the fridge for more flavor. Before you cook the chops let it sit in room temp for 30 min.

Grill or fry the lamb 3-4 min each side. Let it rest 5 min before serving. Sprinkle some dried oregano and tadaaaaaa. You can serve the chops with any side dishes of your desire. I usually make some sort of veggie side or my chopped salad.

My Butter Cup Of Joe

You Need:

Coffee (Organic a must)
MCT oil (I use ONNIT brand)
Kerrygold Unsalted Grass-Fed Butter or Ghee
French press
Blender
Collagen *optional

Prep:

Boil the water, put the amount of coffee you like into the French press, fill it with hot water, let it simmer for 3 min. After transferring everything into the blender, add tablespoon of MCT oil, tablespoon of butter, I usually add my collagen powder in it too, but it's up to you. Pinch of salt is always good so you will stay hydrated.

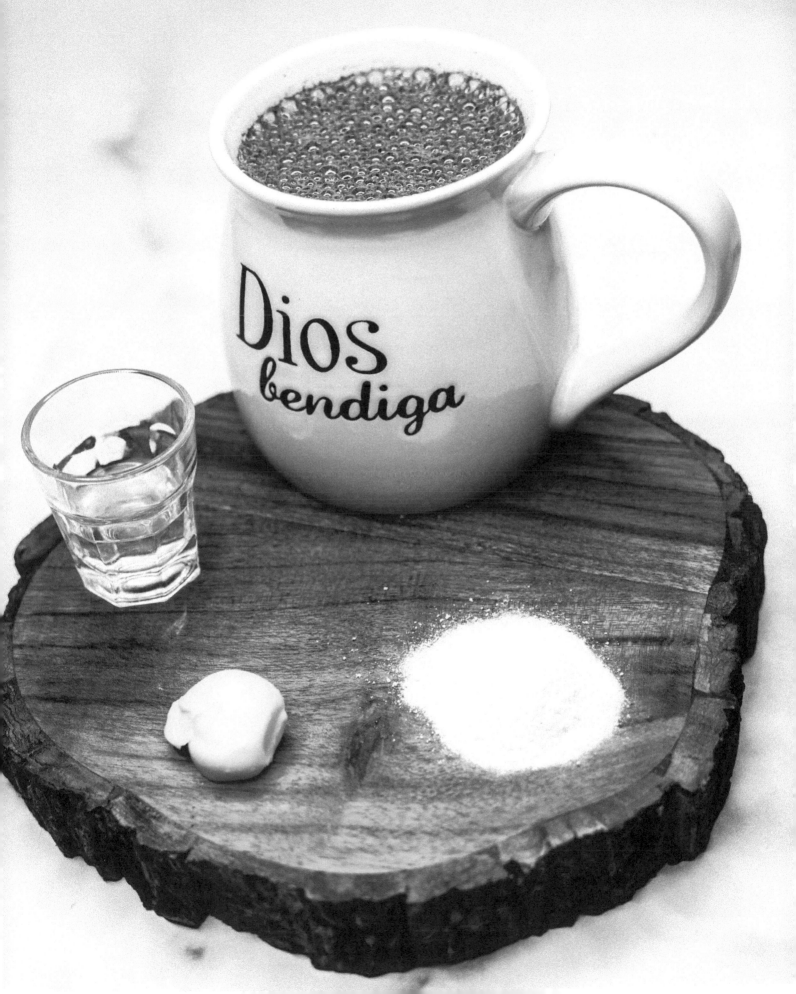

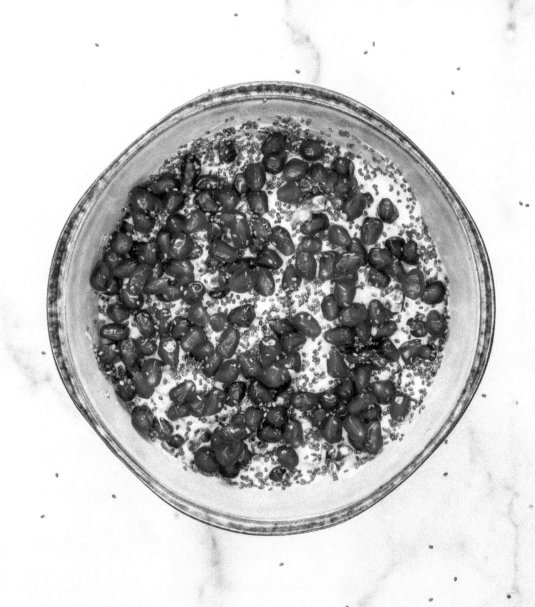

Pom-Yo-Chia

You Need:

1 Cup pomegranate
½ Plain yogurt
1 Teaspoon chia seeds

Prep:

First put the yogurt in a bowl, add the pomegranate seeds and sprinkle the chia seeds. Super easy and super yummy, this is one of my favorite desserts. I don't know if I should call it a dessert. If you mix all of it and leave it in the fridge for a bit, it becomes an amazing pudding, I never have the patience to wait, I just eat it freshly made, but that's also another way of serving. Enjoy!

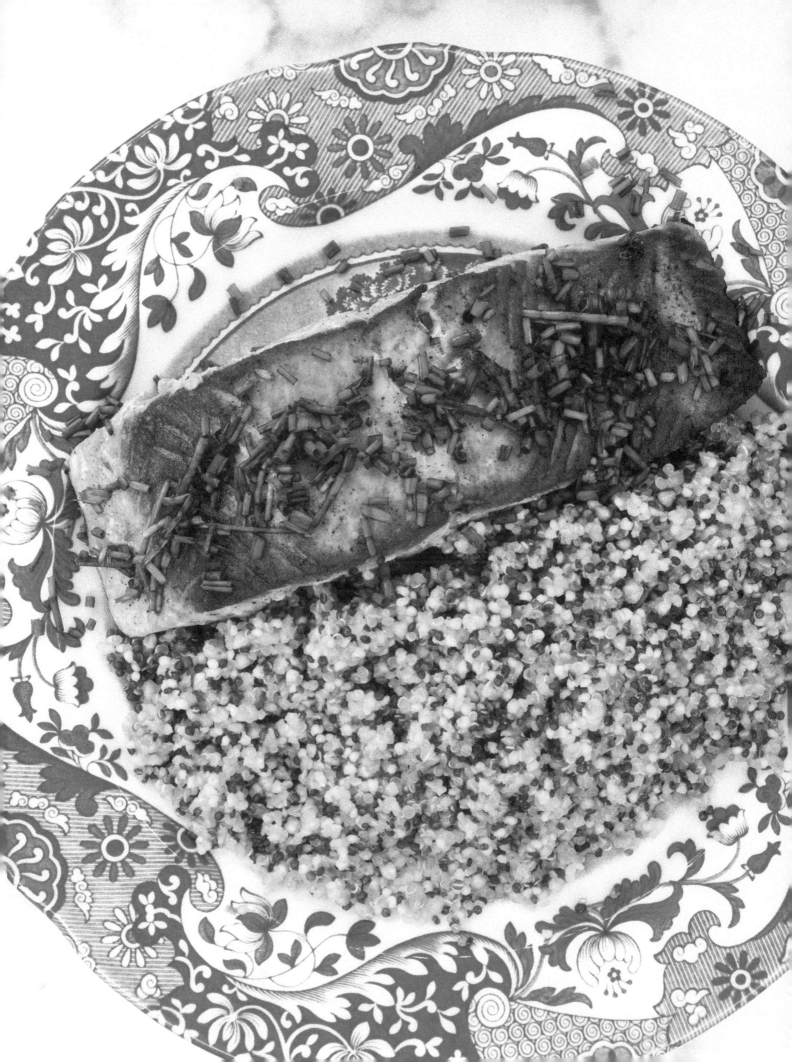

Salmon

You Need:

Wild Salmon
Garlic Powder
¼ cup Soy Sauce
Avocado oil for cooking

Prep:

Rub the salmon with soy sauce and garlic powder and fry it. Serve with any side dish you desire. I told you I cook easy food.

New York Steak

You Need

New york steak (grass-fed, grass-finished)
Olive oil
Soy sauce
Kosher Salt
Black pepper

Prep:

Rub the meat with olive oil, soy sauce, salt and pepper. Let it marinade 30 min, after, cook each side 4 min. for rare to medium rare. Serve with any side desired.

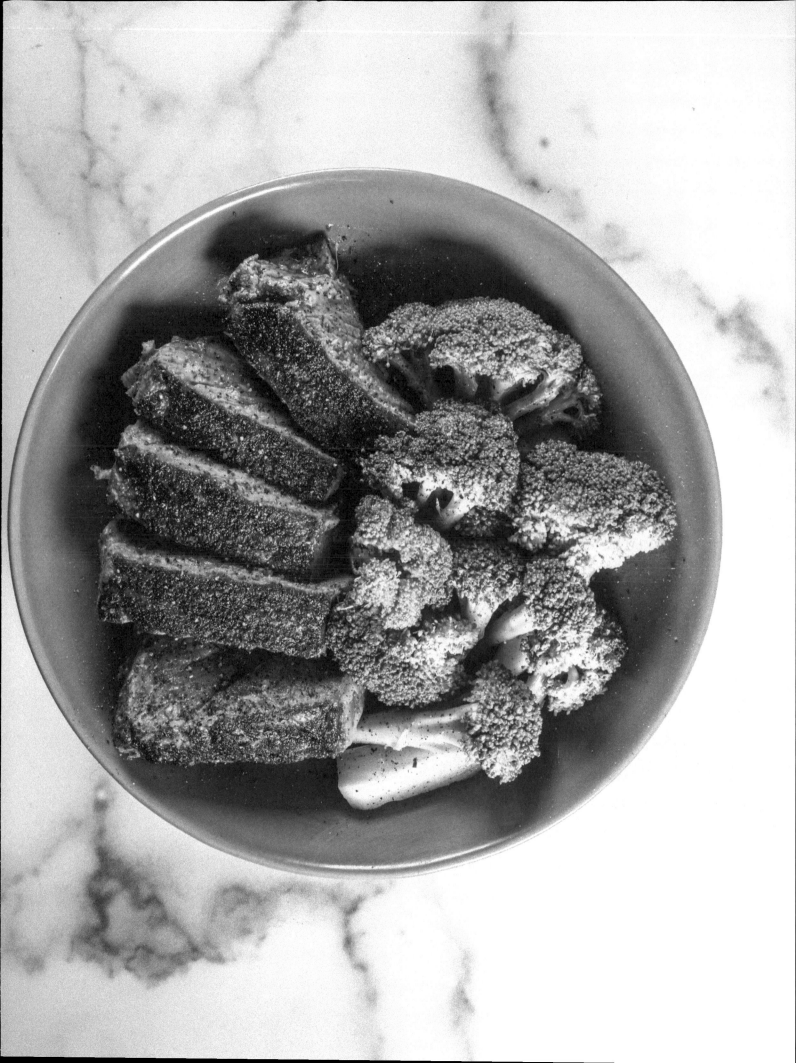

If every individual human body is the embodiment of the sacred land that it belongs to, then our soul is the connection between those lands who complete the circle of the universe. Our souls are like an invisible golden thread that acts as streams to connect the opposite lands together.

I only could explain running into you with the language of poetry and nature. As you and I met randomly on the street, it made me think that the universe had an insane plan for us. You and I, coming from the Anatolian lands or the land of Cybele, "The Mother Goddesses", we carried a common gene in our blood; A powerful sisterhood, an unspeakable language that formed very quickly after we met. We build our own streams that flow wild and free, connecting opposite lands with golden threads having the philosophy of "Wabi-Sabi" in our minds as well as circling and completing layers of experiences in each other's lives.

You had a big impact on my life. Your knowledge and confidence of how women should act and react to situations made me realize my worth, and become a mirror to myself. Your words become my guide and they continue to light my way as they did when I first needed it the most. A healthy mind and a fit body will together create more to our beautiful world, make it fantastic books, artworks, or movies. After being with you for many years, I adopted the values you showed me and now I help others with it too.

Thank you for being yourself, being strong, and lighting up people's way. I am honored to be part of this book as I saw it coming together like a baby from your nurturing nature. Let's keep empowering each other as we keep connecting the streams with the golden thread souls, as you carefully create your land.

Elif Koyuturk

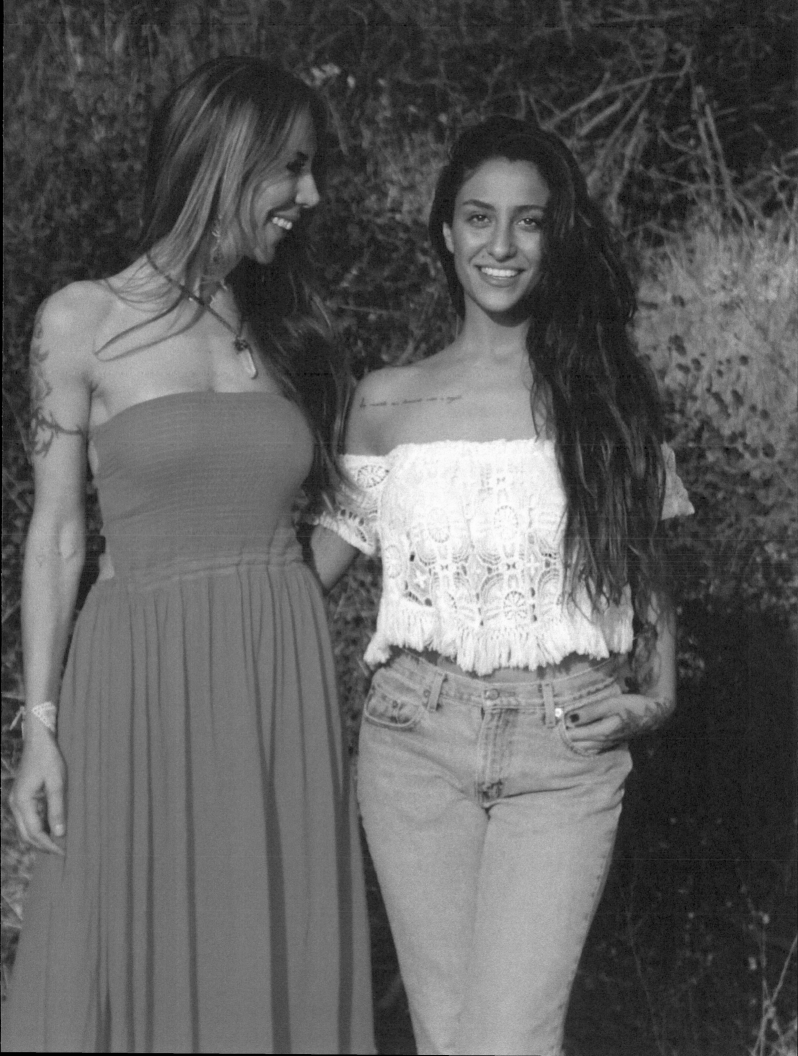

CPSIA information can be obtained
at www.ICGtesting.com
Printed in the USA
BVHW050844090322
630995BV00005B/174